W9-CBP-416

Avalanche

ALSO BY JULIA LEIGH

Novels

Disquiet

The Hunter

Screenplay

Sleeping Beauty

Avalanche

A LOVE STORY

Julia Leigh

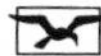

W. W. NORTON & COMPANY
Independent Publishers Since 1923
NEW YORK | LONDON

Avalanche is a work of nonfiction.
Some names and identifying details have been changed.

The author recognizes her shaping of the story may differ from that of other characters depicted in the book.

Printed in the United States of America
First Edition

For information about permission to reproduce selections from this book, write to Permissions, W. W. Norton & Company, Inc., 500 Fifth Avenue, New York, NY 10110

For information about special discounts for bulk purchases, please contact W. W. Norton Special Sales at specialsales@wwnorton.com or 800-233-4830

Manufacturing by RR Donnelley North Harrisonburg
Book design by JAM Design
Production manager: Louise Mattarelliano

ISBN 978-0-393-29276-3

W. W. Norton & Company, Inc.
500 Fifth Avenue, New York, N.Y. 10110
www.wwnorton.com

W. W. Norton & Company Ltd.
Castle House, 75/76 Wells Street, London W1T 3QT

1 2 3 4 5 6 7 8 9 0

Avalanche

For a great many nights I injected myself with an artificial hormone produced in a line of genetically modified Chinese hamster ovary cells. I did this knowing that no matter how hard I hoped, no matter what I tried, chances were I'd never have a child.

My first visit to the IVF clinic was when I was already 38. I was accompanied by Paul, the man I planned to marry and with whom I'd first been in love when I was 19 and he was 23, both of us then studying at the University of Sydney. That same year, it was back in 1989, I wrote a short story that won a student prize. This pleased me because I wanted to be a writer and, more so, because it made me look good in the eyes of my friends. I did keep a copy somewhere but have trouble recalling the exact details—except for the last line, which was "Crazy bitches." The two women of the story were on a bridge in a park and one of them had tossed a baby into the pond below. A passing jogger, a man, had raced in to save the child only to find that it was a doll. At the time of writing that story I had a deeply ambivalent view of motherhood. I scorned women who thought they could only feel fulfilled if they had a child. The first thing the judge said to me at the award ceremony was "I thought you'd be older."

Our relationship began when I bumped into Paul walking from one building to another between lectures. He was wearing a polka-dot shirt and did a double-take: "Hello!" He could be like that—effusive, exuberant, the right side of comic. He was also handsome. More beautiful than handsome. Tall, dark hair, blue eyes, aquiline nose, small full mouth, a Roman. Expressive fine hands. Lady legs. I adored him. But this early love did not last long, it collapsed after a year. The end was his doing, there was no real showdown. He wanted to sleep with other people—as well as with me; he didn't want to be monogamous. This didn't come as a surprise. Early in our courtship he'd taken me aside and said he had something important to tell me: he'd been at a party and had performed cunnilingus on a girl against the living-room wall while everyone was dancing. That was the word he used—cunnilingus—very formal. He wanted to be the first to break the news. The incident did perturb me but in those initial weeks of our relationship, initiatory weeks, I felt like a traveler in a foreign land where it was incumbent on me to observe the strange new local etiquette. It was after we had agreed to the lovers' contract, the body seal, that I couldn't bear the thought of him being intimate with another. A girl was lurking around and the revelation that she had been secretly hurling herself at Paul made me ill. I said he could sleep with the interloper for two weeks. He wanted longer. And so that was it.

We stayed friends. We each fell in and out of love with ten thousand people. Every time I saw him I would be delighted. More than delighted—overjoyed, reconnected. I know exactly how I felt: I witnessed that same feeling the first time I picked up my niece, Elsie, age 2, from day care. This was a long way down the track. About six little ones were sitting in a circle with their teacher, waiting patiently for their parents to arrive. When I entered it took Elsie a split second to realize I was there in her mother's stead—but once she did she leapt up, arms stretched high to the sky, and ran away from her group of playmates, forgetting them forever, rushed toward me.

Paul made me laugh; I made him laugh. We were conspirators. Beneath that was a bone-deep sense of *recognition.*

Yes, I was always slightly jealous of whatever new girlfriend he had; I regarded her with unfriendly close attention. When I was 24 and we were at the first wedding of our peers—a gay wedding, not legal—Paul said we should get back together, get married. I was drunk and turned him down. There's a picture of me in the wedding album—I'm wearing kitten heels, fifties-style black shorts, a men's shirt, and I'm sitting down, unable to stand, my wasted youth, a champagne glass emptying onto the ground. Not long after that wedding Paul met his Irish beloved, a costume designer, and soon they were married and he was a father. He hurried to leave the country.

To this day I know very little about what he was up to in those years away: I never really asked for more than the broad brushstrokes. He worked at an executive level in mortgage finance, earned a good salary. Supported his wife and child. Went on fancy European holidays. He had completely stopped composing music, something at which he had earlier excelled. I recall meeting him once: he made the trip from Dublin to London to see me reading from my first novel at the Southbank Centre. It was a dreary affair cooked up by Australia House to promote Australian literature . . . or maybe I'm remembering it wrong and my publisher organized the night with other Australian writers in their stable. Either way, I felt embarrassed because I was new to the literary world and considered readings an awkward kind of pantomime. I desperately wanted Paul to think well of me, to be impressed, but the circumstances were underwhelming. When the reading had finished we walked together by the river. I noted that under his suit he was wearing the exact same T-shirt he used to wear when we were together. It couldn't have lasted that long so he must have bought a new one: gray marle, with a stick-figure man doing the splits. I was crushed when he said he had to go, didn't ask me to dinner.

In October 2007 I was living in New York, working on a screenplay and a novel. Paul and I reunited. By now he had the marriage and a garland of girlfriends behind him; he was also a loving father to a 12-year-old son. I was 37 with my own trail of tender affections. I received an email announcing he was passing through town. Would I like to meet? He knocked at the door of the miniature studio I was subletting in the West Village. All the chemicals of love spilled through my bloodstream. We spent the day together. Walked around the neighborhood, talked, saw a documentary about mass-produced corn. Talked and talked. Ate and talked and nodded and laughed and stared and smiled and talked and smelled and grinned and I was 19 again, he was 23, and we parted, chaste, my heart thumping, and I realized—joyfully—that it was too late, our soulless souls had flared, whatever doubts I'd ever had about him I no longer wanted to protect myself, I just didn't care.

"OK. Time to be direct. I adore you. I always have and always will whatever happens." He took decisive action. When he returned to Australia he wrote to me from the Southern Highlands, just outside of Sydney, where he now lived in a small house while his ex-wife and son lived in another small house nearby. A warm and civil arrangement. He expressed his fears that our chance may have already been lost; that he had grown dull and hard; that we could hurt one another. He worried about what I wanted: did I really want him or did I just wonder what it might be like to be together? Did I want a child? He promised that there was nothing he would not do for me if we met each other full and open. "Could you bury me? Can you see yourself with me until then?" he asked.

The child, the child. The child was there in that correspondence, nestled in among words of fear and hope and promise. *Our child.* Our beautiful child, our destined child was called forth as a possibility, conjured out of the ether. I told him that yes, I wanted a child very much, and that I did understand the magnitude of that commitment. I no longer wanted to be responsible solely for myself, I wanted to be intimately involved in the care of another. And I also said—it pains me now—that I needed to safeguard "my hard-won creative life." Why was I so quick to add any sort of caveat? Why did I set the two ways of being—motherhood, writing—at odds? The truth, which I knew very well at the time, was that many women had gone before me and found ways to lead a creative life and also be a mother. There were countless prams in countless hallways. It wasn't "rocket science." It wasn't either/or. There was enough space. The universe was expansive. Universe? Old-fashioned. Didn't we live in a multiverse? I could have multiple centers of being; I already had multiple centers of being. Or no center at all. So I wrote to tell all of this to Paul—as best I could—assuaging his anxiety and mine, adopting the tone of someone much wiser than myself, emanating the invincible power of love. I drew strength from the future. From *our child*, the treasured child-to-be. "Darling, darlinger, darlingest," I said. "We only have this one life to live so we are obliged to be magicians."

There's another email worth mentioning. November 6, 2007. That day *The New York Times* ran a story on page 4 titled "A Foul Menace, Ready to Burst Again onto Gaza." It was reported that a LAGOON OF SEWERAGE (I used all caps at the time) had broken through its embankments and flooded an impoverished village. Five died, along with scores of sheep and goats. There was a real threat of another sewerage deluge. It's the only news story on the entire page, I told Paul. That report of abject misery is surrounded by huge ads for luxury goods. Diamond earrings; a zebra print handbag; a Philippe Starck candleholder; three bejeweled rings. So perverse: I suggested we frame it. I can see that even though I was already enthralled with our new-old love I hadn't yet completely lost perspective. No matter how miserable things could ever be for me I was not at risk of *drowning in a lagoon of sewerage.*

Early December. At the airport we kissed for the first time in eighteen years. We went home to my tiny apartment in South Bondi. I showered; we made love. We entered what we called our feral period, lovefucking day and night. It was so much better than when we'd been young. A couple of weeks later he asked "May we marry?"

I said yes without hesitation. The sun exploded then reformed. I remember that instead of an engagement ring he gave me a golden wedding band he'd bought from an antique store in the Southern Highlands; he knew I thought the prestige of a diamond ring was a hoax. I noticed an inscription on the inside of the band. "Oh it's engraved," I said, touched. His face fell in horror: I realized he had never noticed this himself. There was a moment of silent mutual panic. But it was all right; I read the inscription aloud—a jeweler's mark, "18ct Rodd."

I suggested we should be engaged for a year. We decided to marry on the solstice, December 21, 2008. Since we both wanted a child we felt we had to be sure our relationship was truly solid, that it could take the beatings of dirty nappies, dirty dishes, sleeplessness, sexlessness, and whatever else a new baby ensured. Actually, it was a stupid formality. I didn't have time to be cautious. I knew him; I recognized him; I truly loved him. He had offered everything. Our union was *inevitable*. One of my inner eels had slipped loose, an eel that took the guise of reasonable caution but which really was a small wriggling mistrust.

We drove to the highlands for the New Year. On the radio there was a discussion about the death threats once made against a Danish newspaper cartoonist who had unfavorably depicted Mohammad. In response, we decided to devise the most offensive, the most grossly offensive cartoon image we could possibly think of. I took pleasure in our playful transgression. My sweet husband: the same breed of monster. It was certain he would never bore me—and wasn't this the Holy Grail of marriage . . . or so I'd been told. (Misinformed.) We spent a cozy New Year's Eve together; we cooked a meal and watched Ermanno Olmi's *I Fidanzati*, *The Fiancés*, on DVD. He wore a sea-green Chinese silk dressing gown that I'd found for him earlier that day in the local antique store; it was more like a wonder emporium than a store. For myself I'd picked out some hand-embroidered oyster silk shorts. My predilection for soft silky clothing turned out to be something we didn't share: he thought it slippery. When I used to wear my UGG boots, tracksuit pants, and a pink silk T-shirt around the house he'd ruefully shake his head and say, "You look like a jockey." That New Year's Eve, laying my head on the warm hairy pillow of his chest, I was a tiny baby. At long last, rested.

We bought a bottle of Cointreau and called it kissing syrup. Over breakfast he'd play love songs like Nick Cave's "Sweetheart Come" or "Do You Realize??" by The Flaming Lips. When we listened to The Beatles' "Come Together" we'd loudly interject, so the lyrics became "Come *Almost* Together." He gave me a golden compass. I was erotically charged when he would help me zip up the back of my dress. We shared all our "elective affinities." And our vulnerabilities—lovers' currency. One day we made a visit back to campus especially to kiss in the stacks of the library. We had our own names for local landmarks. I called him my Gentle Liege, my Ur-Prince, my Anarchist Master. He was also known as Captain Frolic, the Resplendent Quetzal, and the Magnificent Pigeon. I bought his favorite foods at the grocery store. He gave me the name Cheese Prices because I would despair at the cost of a block of cheese, calculating I needed to sell five books per block. We counted the days since we'd reunited at the airport—that was Day 1, we reset the calendar. Each night we'd give thanks for the day together; each morning we'd greet one another on waking. There were minor skirmishes at the border . . . and he would call an Emergency Meeting that involved him lying flat on the floor and I would lie on top of him and we'd talk things through that way, nose to nose. It was summer so we swam together and took walks along the Bondi cliff tops. I pointed out an avalanche in a white curl of wave breaking against the shore. When we passed a man coming in the opposite direction with a baby strapped to his chest Paul squeezed my hand. We dared to discuss baby names. For some reason, I think because he already had a son, we only talked about girls' names. I said I liked names ending in "ia." "Indicia," he suggested. "And she'll know she's met the right person when they ask 'Of what?' " I didn't like it that much, thought it too tricksy, as if it belonged in a Thomas Pynchon novel, but we kept it as an option, a precious placeholder. Returning from a business trip, Paul bought a little teddy bear in a pink top at the airport. Whenever either of us would travel alone that teddy bear would go in the suitcase.

Our child. In February 2008 we made our first visit to the IVF clinic. There was the not insignificant matter of a vasectomy to deal with, a procedure Paul had undergone not long after the birth of his son. Our plan, our hope, was that a vasectomy reversal would work and I'd fall pregnant naturally, wouldn't need further intervention—but just in case the reversal failed or I had problems then we wanted to ensure we were in good hands. I went online to compare the success-rate claims of the two Sydney clinics I'd heard the most talk about. I didn't keep notes at the time but today I went back to the same clinic websites and looked at their information. I figure the statistics haven't radically altered: if anything the chances of IVF working have only improved over time. For women aged between 35 and 39, using their own eggs, one clinic claimed a live birth rate per embryo transfer (fresh and frozen) of 28 percent. A transfer is a procedure where an embryo is placed in the uterus or fallopian tubes; the embryo can be fresh or it can have been thawed following freezing. When I looked at the second clinic I found it presented its data differently. It used a narrower age range; didn't give exact percentages in numerical form but instead relied on a visual graph with columns per age group; and it counted only fresh transfers, not frozen. The graph showed that for women using their own eggs between 37 and 39 years there was a live birth rate of around 22 percent for each fresh embryo transfer. On the same graph the natural conception rate for a woman aged 37 to 39 was 10 percent. A direct comparison of success rates between the two clinics wasn't possible—perhaps by design. And there was nowhere else I could turn to for clarity: in Australia data about the IVF industry has been collected but the success rates that identify specific clinics are not released to the public.

Back then, right at the beginning, I had an uneasy response to the so-called statistics. I told myself: each human body is a mystery; there are too many factors that distinguish one 38-year-old from another. What if one woman had only one ovary? What if another had endometriosis? Didn't they drag down the overall probabilities of success? An aggregate figure was not convincing. My own chances would surely be better (this was the irrational leap). Paul had another name for me: Pollyanna Juggernaut. Pollyanna was determined to look on the bright side, plow ahead. She would not, could not, countenance the abyss. I always liked Pollyanna Juggernaut: she would lead the troops to battle.

What actually swung our choice of clinic was not the data but a personal recommendation from a trusted friend, someone I'd known since high school and who was diligent by nature, always doing a lot of homework before taking a step ahead. She'd tried one place and had no luck, then moved on. She recommended a man whom I shall call Dr. Rogers. "I didn't like him," she said, "but he's the guy who got me pregnant." Dr. Rogers, it turned out, according to his web profile, had an expertise in male infertility. So I went ahead and fixed an appointment.

The clinic was in the central business district, somewhere I'd largely avoided since graduation from law school. For me, a trip to the city had the novelty of a trip to the Big Smoke. We took the elevator to the fifth floor, both having made an effort to be well dressed, citified, as if stepping into the clinic together was as symbolic a first step in marriage as any state-sanctioned union. Heads in the waiting room did not turn. This was a temple of discretion. No one expected or wanted to be here. Immediately I noticed the wallpaper was neither girl-pink nor boy-blue but a considerate shade of yellow. The magazines on the low tables were up to date. Paul and I held hands (who reached out their hand first for comfort, to comfort, I don't know). Dr. Rogers was friendly. It must have been the kind of appointment he looked forward to—a new couple, committed to having a child together, glowing with an undimmed hope. We hung off his every word. What we were chiefly there for was to talk about reversing the vasectomy. Ah, the vasectomy! Dr. Rogers reached into his drawer and pulled out a laminated flipbook of gruesome surgical photos. He regaled us with a detailed description of what would need to be done. Paul would have a general anesthetic. The tubes that carry the sperm from the testes along with other ejaculate are called the vasa (collective) or vas (singular). The vasa—left side and right side—had been snipped and the doctor would find the two ends of each snipped tube or vas, remove the scar tissue, and attempt to rejoin the ends. As a result, the sperm that Paul was currently producing and which couldn't find its way up the vasa would be able to flow free. A feat of irrigation engineering worthy of a Balinese subak master. A small mystery was solved for me: the sperm he had been producing with snipped tubes had just died on the spot and been reabsorbed by the body, it hadn't gone anywhere. Even if the tubes were successfully rejoined—the long length of time between the vasectomy and the reversal diminished our odds—it wasn't guaranteed the sperm would return. And if it didn't? Dr. Rogers explained that during the procedure they'd also take a significant amount of sperm and freeze it so that it could later be used for multiple treatment cycles. And if we wanted, at any future time, fresh sperm could be taken straight from the testes, during another minor operation.

Testes: I felt squeamish; I sensed Paul was embarrassed, he didn't like being in a position where another man was so passionate about cutting into his balls. The doctor then turned his attention to me. He asked if I smoked (no) or drank (in moderation) and assessed my body mass index (healthy). Age? 38. "Hmmm, that's generally fine," he said, "but I don't want to see you back here in two years' time." Back in two years' time? *What are you talking about?* In Dr. Rogers's office, at his suggestion of a potential return visit in two years' time, I remember being a little offended.

"I've been pregnant before," I jumped in. "Twice. In my twenties. Two terminations." It was a good thing, I thought, it raised my chances. If I'd been pregnant before then odds were I could be pregnant again. I wasn't one of those unlucky women who belatedly discover some serious problem with their uterus. I have never, not even for one second, regretted those terminations—not even now. Dr. Rogers picked up his pen. He drew a simple graph. Natural fertility on the vertical axis, age on the horizontal, starting at age 25 and running to 50. As a woman aged her fertility dropped, the downward slope became precipitous. He tried to impress on me the fact that my early pregnancies had less bearing on my current situation than I thought. They were a lifetime ago. Nor did he give much weight to the fact that my sister had easily fallen pregnant or that my mother had a late menopause. As soupy as the statistics were, as malleable, a woman's age was a key determinant in her chances of "taking home a baby."

He ordered a battery of tests. We thanked him and left. Signed some paperwork at the front desk. Paid by credit card. We hardly spoke in the elevator, held our breath. Pollyanna Juggernaut deserted me. I was tiny. Thrown. Out on the street, Paul put his arm around my shoulders, pulled me close. I was thinking: I hope the reversal works; I hope my test results are OK; please, please, please, I never want to come back here.

There's a different graph Dr. Rogers could have drawn that first day in the clinic. Most IVF cycles fail, or to be more precise, most *assisted reproduction* fails. The best source of statistics I've found is an independent study by the National Perinatal and Statistics Unit within the University of New South Wales. Published in September 2015, the report analyzes data collected from all assisted reproduction technology clinics in Australia and New Zealand in the year 2013. It shows, among other things, that of 71,516 treatment cycles only 18.2 percent resulted in a live birth. Regardless the age of the patient, regardless the exact variant of treatment, most cycles failed. So Dr. Rogers could have marked treatment failure on the vertical axis and a woman's age on the horizontal. It's an industry predicated on failure. The true graph depicts a mountain with one face Hope and the other Despair.

I did my blood tests. Since I was young I've had a phobia of needles. My mother thinks it stems from an early childhood visit to the doctors when I yanked my arm away mid-procedure. What a mess. Once at the university medical center I was settling my account after a blood test and I heard a loud bang. I came to lying on the ground with someone holding two fingers in front of my face, asking me to count them. When I'd fainted I'd accidentally swiped the receptionist's large intercom system off her desk and onto the floor—that accounted for the bang I'd heard. I was dragged by the feet through the waiting room into a corridor. It was nearing the end of the day so a kind doctor drove me home. Still, it doesn't seem to me hysterical to have an intense dislike of a needle piercing my vein and draining blood from my body. It's creepy. Also, I have bad veins, reluctant veins—which means that sometimes it takes more than one go to strike gold. (I'm so phobic I even cringe at typing the word *vein*.) I bruise; I get blood blisters; I break out in a rash. In the course of my treatment I did close to a hundred blood tests, probably more. I developed a strict routine: heat pack, lie down, left arm first, turn my head to the side and let the tears fall. Symptom: I would sink into a disproportionate state of vulnerability, the tears would rise unbidden as I resigned myself to that vulnerability. Needle out. Pressing my finger on my vein to staunch the prick was completely disgusting to me. "Please don't show me the vial of blood, just read out my name and birth date." I never found it easy.

I became very interested in what age a woman had her first child. Just as I used to try to figure out when an author had published their first novel now I sought to compare myself with new mothers. The point of comparison was not to do better but to get a feel for the lay of the land. To gauge what was not impossible. Again, the persuasive illogic: if she could do it at age 38, 39, 40, 41, 42, 43, 44, then so could I. My sources were various. First, there were the anecdotal accounts among friends and friends-of-friends. Dozens of women in my broad circle had their babies late. One friend naturally fell pregnant at 45 and then at 47, thanks to freakishly good genes and—according to her—copious shots of wheatgrass. Later, when I began to confide that I'd started treatment, I would invariably be reassured and provided with an example or two of a recent success story. The media, too, was full of good news. It seemed that every second day a celebrity in her forties was having a baby. I gratefully swallowed the evidence.

The druids in the lab read my blood and reported back. Dr. Rogers talked us through the results. Amongst a raft of other things I was all clear for hepatitis, HIV, rubella, syphilis. My thyroid was fine. A full blood count didn't present any problems. My iron was on the low side, as was my B12, but nothing dreadful. My progesterone and estrogen levels were normal. A genetic test showed I didn't carry cystic fibrosis. Nor did I have any sperm antibodies. The pelvic ultrasound concluded "No pelvic abnormality is detected at this examination."

The doctor had also tested my follicle stimulating hormone level. The FSH test was supposed to give insight into the remaining number of eggs I had—but it could not tell me anything about the quality of those eggs. FSH is a hormone produced by the pituitary gland that plays a regulatory role in both stimulating the growth of follicles and letting the body know when it is time to ovulate. A follicle is the sac of fluid that surrounds a developing egg. As a woman ages and her stockpile of eggs diminishes it takes more FSH to produce an egg. The correlation seems to be that the more effort it takes, the higher the FSH reading, the lower the egg supply or "ovarian reserve." A result of 8.1 was deemed by Dr. Rogers to be "reasonable." Sitting there in his room I had the sense that all augured well: if the vasectomy reversal worked then a natural pregnancy wasn't out of the question.

I nurtured this belief that I would fall pregnant naturally. Why be nervous? If it really were true that only 10 percent of women aged 38 fell pregnant naturally (and I had my doubts) then I would be among the *millions* of women in the world who had once upon a time fitted that description. Pollyanna Juggernaut could do amazing things with the figures. I would be one of the lucky ones, an exception. After all, didn't I have a track record for beating the odds? When I was 27 I was diagnosed with a tumor in my left lung. It wasn't possible to do a biopsy at the time of the bronchoscopy, there was too high a risk of bleeding. Because of the central location of the tumor, the whole lung (and lymph nodes) had to be immediately removed. Lung carcinoma is the leading cause of cancer death. I had the operation and waited days for the result. When the registrar told me the amazing news—it was a carcinoid, not carcinoma—I just nodded like I'd been told it was three o'clock in the afternoon. He said I was a hard lady to please. This was because usually less than 1 percent of all tumors in the lung are carcinoids, a relatively slow-growing neuroendocrine tumor. I was on morphine but really I was so blasé because I had never taken on board the known likelihood of carcinoma. Before surgery I had willfully disconnected from the probabilities. In my critical state they weren't helpful.

In the public imagination—as I perceive it—there's a qualified sympathy for IVF patients, not unlike that shown to smokers who get lung cancer. Unspoken: "You signed up for it, so what did you expect . . . ?"

Nearing the end of my treatment it became harder and harder to kid myself that I was lucky, exceptional, or altogether outside the realm of statistics. The real reason I didn't want to know about the IVF numbers was that I was desperate.

Our probationary year disappeared. During that time I decided to put up my hand to direct my screenplay. It was a long shot the film would get made since I'd never directed any sort of film before. My novel was published: I was happy with the reception. For Paul's birthday I gave him a word. "To smund: when a woman, a wife, lays her length upon a man, her husband, and with slow loving sinuous movements caresses, presses her soft warm breasts against his chest." One day we were walking home from the grocery store, and I said something very homey, something like, "When we get home I'll put the potatoes on." "Will you, Mrs. McGillicuddy?" he replied. It was a sublime moment: the birth of Mr. and Mrs. McGillicuddy, there on the footpath, fully grown, the long-married homey couple, the cardigan wearers, the ones who put the potatoes on. After that we often used to call each other Mr. or Mrs. McGillicuddy, it became one of our fondest endearments. In November 2008 Paul underwent his vasectomy reversal. And on the December solstice, as agreed, Mr. and Mrs. McGillicuddy were married.

Scene from a marriage: Night in the highlands, we had a fight and he ordered me out of the house. I had nowhere to go. Because I'd never learned to drive I wasn't able to get in the car and drive back to Sydney. I walked into town and found a pub, closed, where the staff were having last drinks. Knocked loudly on the door. I tried not to cry as I apologized for disturbing them, asked to pay for a room. Upstairs, lying in the narrow bed, fully dressed, I took out my phone. Paul had left many messages. I thought about switching it off before letting him know I was safe but I also had an urgent desire to hear his voice. Heartbroken, remorseful, he begged to come and pick me up and I agreed.

That is how in my 39th year I came to make love, for the first time in my life, with a deep desire to physically conceive, to procreate, to make a baby. It was so beautiful. Crossing over into one another, imagining the pleasure of orgasm as a kind of nurturing magic field for the moment of conception. A molecular union. Lovefucking for *our child*. And today I remain thankful for those experiences. But it was impossible to sustain, that keenly pitched sacred pleasure. As month after month passed and I did not fall pregnant the obligation to make love on the days around my time of ovulation became wearisome. One month Paul had a conference in a country town at "that time" and I traveled up there to be with him so that we could try. We stayed in a chintzy bed'n'breakfast. I can't remember exactly how it happened but we were meant to make love in the morning before our early departure, at around 6 a.m. That was the opportune window. I had no genuine bodily desire whatsoever but was amenable to a pragmatic quickie. Paul tried—with no luck. Too much pressure. A situation that for the two of us was equal parts frustrating, humiliating, chintzy, and bathetic. It cast a pall over the day. He didn't like—and nor did I—how our lovefucking had become so colored by the desire for a child, as if that were now its sole purpose. We agreed we'd try to take the pressure off and not be so focused on my menstrual cycle. All that meant was we didn't talk about it while I remained acutely aware of exactly how near or far I was to ovulation.

There came a day when I reached a sunken crossroad. My film—miraculously—got its coveted green light, the full financing was committed. What to do: how could I direct a feature film and become pregnant at the same time? The stress of making the film would be bad for the baby; potential health complications would be bad for the film. Which-way, which-way, which-way. Where were the omens? After a week of sleepless nights I told Paul I wanted us to stop trying to get pregnant, I said I would take precautions for six months until the film was shot and I was in the edit. He was disappointed and though he didn't say as much I worried he saw my choice as a betrayal. It made him wary, and wariness, in retrospect, is poison in a union. Even if he'd tried to persuade me to drop the film I don't think I would have done so. Sometimes I wish I had been less fearful.

I completely immersed myself in making the film and I neglected my husband. There were repercussions.

"You're so busy I might as well not be here." One night during the shoot he repeated his trick of ordering me out of the house (at the time we were living in a new apartment we'd bought together). A few days later he left to spend time with his son who was now 14 and living in Ireland with his mother. The film wrapped: he didn't call. On the day of his return we had a fight. His anger was frightening and intolerable. I took half of my stuff and moved back to my old place which was just around the corner. *I can't stand it!* There followed a complicated tangle of emotions—hurts, desires, everything else. Bamboozling at the time. Two people in love and at odds. A Gordian knot would have been child's play. I'm not sure I could ever explain it. He said he didn't sign up for me putting my career ahead of everything else, he said I was blind to how my work bled into our lives and obscured all the good things. He wanted more balance. A few weeks later he issued me with legal papers for a full property settlement through the family law courts, to be effective immediately. He wanted the title deed to our new home transferred into solely his name: he'd pay out my share. He wanted to undo all our joint bank accounts and other assets, a complete financial separation. In other words, a divorce. But he refused to call it a divorce. He wanted us to live together "under two roofs." He wanted a moratorium on talking about a family. A moratorium! For how long? Indefinite. He'd pilfered the word "moratorium" from one of the couples counselors, the one who gave us a book that said there was a finite number of possible types of relationship, something like 1,392 or maybe 3,921. Then Paul modified his position and said we could "shuttle between the houses till the baby comes." Topsy-turvy. I thought the property settlement was such a sniveling low demand that ipso facto it warranted divorce. We signed the legal papers in my lawyer's office. I was in tears. That night he came over to my place and we slept together.

Why are you writing this, Rat-wife? Rat-patient. Hey, Queen of the Rats, why?

I guess it's common sense but I sincerely believe in the truth of what I'm writing and at the very same time I know Paul would shape a different story. What's more, I know my own next sentence could turn this way or that.

We reconciled. Beloved singular man, wondrous sea creature, hand-holder—I forgave him everything and vowed to do better in his eyes. Mr. and Mrs. McGillicuddy went back to the clinic. A sperm test showed the vasectomy reversal had failed. The initial sperm flow post-op had been "respectable"—said the doctor—but the test now confirmed a zero sperm count. No sperm. If we wanted to proceed we would have no choice but to begin IVF using the sperm frozen during Paul's operation. Neither of us asked for how long Paul had been without sperm, it seemed discourteous, impossible to know. (A good question: why didn't we test it earlier?) Part of me was pleased—if the reason I hadn't already fallen pregnant was because of low or no sperm flow then that problem could be rectified. What was scary was my own ovarian reserve. My FSH level was retested and it had held steady. Another marker for ovarian reserve was an AMH test. Anti-Müllerian hormone is a hormone secreted by very early ovarian follicles. The clinic ran the test and analyzed the results in their own lab. Like the FSH test, this test could not tell me anything about the quality of my eggs. Nor was the test conclusive: on the upside, I was informed there had been several reported cases of women with undetectable levels of AMH who had fallen pregnant. My level came back as 6.1—which was fractionally better than average for a woman my age. Ovarian reserve diminishes over time: that was the golden rule. When I was tested again in 2012 my level had gone up to 8.3. Alice in Wonderland. I asked Dr. Rogers how that was possible. He shrugged it off. He said a woman of 25 had a level of 50; it was all relative; my reserve was low. I should be glad, he said, the clinic would treat me. It seemed that only a veil of science shrouded the vast mystery.

The doctor didn't try to sugarcoat things, he said he was happy to proceed, all my retested bloods and ultrasound were fine but my age—40—was a problem. He gave me an approximate 20 percent chance of success. Thank you, thank you. I was so grateful, so willing. I didn't hesitate for a moment to abandon Mother Nature. He filled out a consent form for Paul and me to sign that specified our treatment. Ran us through the costs. I played my inner trick of pretending it was all Monopoly money. He checked his watch, smiled kindly, inclined his head toward the door.

If I were devout I would paint exquisite ex-votos on small tin sheets in a Mexican style, illustrating the miracle of IVF conception. A woman with her legs in stirrups. And floating in the surgery theater a little cloud, and in that cloud a sperm nosing into an egg, or perhaps an eight-celled embryo implanting into a red-lined womb. I'd go into churches and pin wax effigies of sprouting ovaries to the wall, in the same way the faithful pin up effigies of their ailing arms and legs.

We never made it back to the clinic together. We scheduled appointments, we were ready to begin treatment, but more than once—at the very last minute—Paul changed his mind. I got the blame for falling asleep at 2 a.m. on a day we were due to begin. We had been up all night talking about our future as parents, he was worried he would be stuck holding the baby, he was worried he was too old. I did my best to assure him all would be fine, better than fine, a joy, a gift . . . but I was bone-tired and soon begged off to sleep. When I woke up Paul told me he was canceling the cycle. He said that if we'd been talking about my work in the early hours of the morning I would have managed to stay awake. He was unsure, he wanted to wait. *Wait!* I felt like I had been stabbed—and wanted to stab him in turn—but I needed his permission and did my best to persuade him to *please* reconsider. Nothing worked. I was a hopeless supplicant.

Things fell apart. Fall down, get back up, fall down. Stay down, duck for cover. It was a long, sad, immensely difficult time for both of us. He said I was relegating "Us" to my insistent desire for a child. I couldn't bear his deliberate procrastinating, his brooding, his rages. The weight of his reproach. My friends and family despaired for me; his friends and family despaired for him. But we were not entirely sad—that was our problem. Our relationship didn't fade out . . . it was syncopated, tender—terrible. So many small things were quietly wonderful. We both sincerely claimed to love one another more than we'd ever loved anyone before, we told ourselves ours were only the best intentions.

My film was selected to be "In Competition" at the Festival de Cannes. The experience was intense and marvelous and I couldn't have survived it without Paul by my side. The night of the screening was also his birthday. At the after-party, held on a beach, he stripped off his tuxedo and went for a swim. Emerging from the water he was radiant. That was in May 2011—but we slid downhill through June and by July we had drafted divorce papers. Over a year had passed since our separation around the time of the property settlement and a formal divorce could now be granted. The paperwork wasn't signed and sent to the family court until October. I sent it in: Paul told me he had started sleeping with other people. Our body seal was broken.

And still, and yet, and don't let go, even after we were officially divorced we continued to see one another. In February 2012 we planned a weekend away at his friend's beach house down the coast, he said we would go there to "create something new together." My hope, as always, was that it would only take a tiny breakthrough and our relationship would crystallize, a slow process culminating in a sudden and unpredictable transformation. We ate fish'n'chips, drank wine, watched DVDs. It poured with rain. When I said "I love you" he flinched. "Why say that now!" "Because we're sitting on the couch, nothing special." Nothing special: nothing worked. Nothing worked. Nothing within me worked. We failed to understand one another deeply. I've revisited that weekend a thousand times. Reenacted—rewritten every conversation, every stillborn attempt at open-hearted conversation. An endless restoration. That was the weekend when we did truly divorce, when even the McGillicuddys had to call it a day. I was grateful to Paul for one thing: we agreed that if we were to irrevocably part he would allow me to use his frozen sperm and go ahead with being a single mother. He knew I didn't want to use a stranger's sperm; he knew how old I was; he knew how I'd found myself in my predicament. I would take full financial responsibility and he could be involved in co-parenting as little or as much as he liked. Since we had been friends for so long—twenty-three years—we felt we could maintain harmony in the future. *Our child* had taken root. I believed I would forever be fond of Paul. He was tattooed under my skin.

I was happy to be a single mother. If the choice was between not being a mother and being a single mother then I had no qualms. Again, millions of women around the world had been or were single mothers, not all by choice—granted. I have several friends who reached the same impasse and made a different and difficult decision. They couldn't see how they would be happy as a single mother, how they could manage the financial pressures, the squeeze of time, the sole responsibility. Some thought that it wouldn't be best for the baby, that a child needed more than one parent, that the bond between a single mother and child could curdle or suffocate. Other friends were perfectly content not being parents; childlessness didn't bother them in the slightest. "Why do it to yourself?" a male friend asked me. He was single, mid-forties, without a child but patiently hoping for a family.

My 42nd birthday passed without celebration. In March 2012 I arranged to visit Paul at home because I needed his signature on a new consent form. Same as before. Our most recent form had expired, each was only good for six months. It was so strange to be standing in the living room, looking at the sofa and rug we had bought together, the chairs we'd upholstered, the framed map on the wall that was an exact replica of the map on my own living-room wall, an Operational Navigation Chart of the South Atlantic Ocean, a map I'd pinned up wherever I'd lived ever since I first came across it over a decade ago. My period was due and I was prepared to begin treatment. For the past couple of weeks I had been slowly gathering strength, adding pregnancy multivitamins to my iodine-folate pill (I'd been on that for ages); cutting down my coffee; doing more exercise; talking to a counselor about proceeding alone. I'd been gathering strength and weeping and weeping. Paul refused to sign the consent form. He announced he had changed his mind. He didn't think I should be a mother; I was too selfish; I didn't know how to love. "You had no commitment to my happiness." What he needed was a clean break. "I'm a decent man who wants nothing more than to live and love simply with family at the center of my life." *Plunge into the deep circular pit.* He tried to bundle me out the door, took hold of me, and I scratched him, hard, broke his skin. I refused to leave, sat down on the sofa. He threatened to call the police and then left. I waited for him to return. I thought about taking a knife to the sofa, ripping it open, ripping my leg open. When he got back he said that earlier that morning, in anticipation of my visit, he had called my parents for their advice. My mother had agreed with him.

Was it true! Outside on the street I called my mother and she confirmed that yes, she didn't think I should be a mother. "And anyway, how would you get to the hospital on your own?" I told her that I would never speak to her again. Then I called one of my sisters. We have long experience with our mother's Honest Tourette's. My sister called my mother, my mother called me back. She didn't think I should be a mother, not with him as the father. I hung up. Mothers and daughters—not always sunshine stories. She never really got on board with my IVF: she thought it a bad idea and because she is so forthright, never insincere, she couldn't fake support. My father took the same view. With wax in my ears I reassured myself that making babies in the lab was virtually unknown in their generation, hence the cool reaction. All updates went through my sisters. In the last months my mother softened and sent kind messages, chicken soup. After one particular disappointment, the latest in a long chain of disappointments, she reminded me of how surprised she'd been when I came home from high school one day and informed her I'd won the cross-country race. "I asked you how you did it and do you remember what you said? 'I pass them on the hills when I'm crying.'"

Whatever was left of my dignity I threw in the bin. I wrote to Paul and apologized for losing my temper. I said I completely accepted our marriage was over. I asked if he could look past his immediate pain and imagine himself in six months' time, in a year's time, happy and vital. Probably with a new love. The choice was his—unquestionably—but could he reconsider with an open heart? I said it was rare that we ever faced such a stark complex decision, so rare for the Fates to reveal themselves. Out of our relationship could come a beautiful childbeing. His life would only be enriched, not ruined. To no avail: he remained unmoved. Still, I was convinced that—after the worst of the bitter pain of divorce had eased—the blood would drain from his eyes and he'd see clearly. Just as before, on so many occasions, I'd seen him burn with fury and then make amends.

I'm an expert at make-believe. *Our child* was not unreal to me. It was not a real child but also it was not unreal. Maybe a better way to say it is that the unknown unconceived had been an inner presence. A desired and nurtured inner presence. Not real but a singular presence in which I had radical faith. A presence that could not be substituted or replaced.

My sleep was infected. I had dreams of searching in frustration for clothes that mysteriously vanished; a golden necklace, opera length, which at 10 cm intervals was broken up with small old-fashioned watch faces; a foul image of biting into a hamburger with a giant blood clot at its center. A nightmare in which Paul came to the door and I saw that he was cradling a dead toddler in his arms. He wasn't smug or victorious, instead he looked at me as if he had only just realized he'd made a terrible, terrible mistake. In that dream my main concern was not to lose my composure, not to unnerve him, because I was holding the hand of another child by my side whom I had to protect.

I could have walked away there and then and used unknown donor sperm from the clinic's sperm bank. That sperm would have already cleared the three-month quarantine period required for any donated sperm. Quarantine is an industry standard in order to guard against HIV and other transmissible diseases. But in the IVF world we all have our parameters, our personal lines in the sand. At least we do when we start out, before the harsh desert winds cut across the dunes. (And some resile from starting out altogether: I heard of a German writer who told her audience that children created through IVF were *Halbwesen*, "twilight creatures," "half-human, half-artificial I-don't-know-whats.") My own parameter was that I couldn't face using a stranger's sperm. I wanted to have a special personal bond with the father of my child. Also, I harbored doubts about anonymous sperm because I figured the donors self-declared their medical history, filled out forms, and that there was very little if any fact-checking, double-checking, very little investigation of that medical history. I was especially concerned about things undetectable in the blood. At heart, I wasn't ready to abandon *our child.* Couldn't face the grief, I suppose. Doubled grief: lost marriage, lost childling. I envied the widows—innocent—whereas I was complicit in my loss. I know a friend who would shrug her shoulders: when she was in her early forties and single she went straight to the sperm bank, did one egg collection, and on her second transfer with a frozen embryo fell pregnant, gave birth to a healthy baby boy. Her life was transformed, filled with love.

I asked again for Paul's frozen sperm. And again. He told me it was too late, I'd had my chance, I'd blown it: "Sillybilly." A couple of months later, when Paul was on holiday, he invited me to join him in Shanghai. An invitation, an opening. What bravery. I read the email, my heart leapt, flared. *All the chemicals of love spilled through my bloodstream.* Imagine: lying in his arms again; his smell; his face softening, losing its edges. Imagine: beginning again. Standing very close to one another. Holding hands. But by morning I was trembling. Hadn't we always been in love and hadn't we tried, and tried, and hadn't we never managed to make things work. So I wrote to say it would be better if I saw him when he returned. He said I was blind to the only truly great thing in my life, "Us," and that his deep sadness was due to my doubting, my hovering, my lack of trust. Soon we were in touch again. He drafted the letter that he wished I'd written him, my mea culpa, from me to him. If I'd been able to write that mea culpa he would have forgiven me everything, he said, but as I hadn't, he was turning away. A month later he met his new partner—or re-met, since they had known one another as teenagers. I was happy because she was older, closer to 50, and had two primary-school-age children of her own: she wouldn't want his frozen sperm. I thought that now Paul was happy, head over heels, we could move into a kind of brotherly-sisterly après-love. They hadn't been together long before I bumped into them at the art gallery. I saw him first, alone. He was glowing. A new shirt, new jeans, new haircut. He greeted me warmly, we hugged. Had a polite chat, parted. When I moved into the next room I watched him kneel down and raise a young girl onto his shoulders. He glanced up at me with the chill dead-eyes of a shark. The two-headed man-girl went to stand alongside a woman and her son and they gazed into a large mirror, an Anish Kapoor work, admiring a distorted family portrait. The flow of the exhibition was such that I had to walk directly past them. On the way I went up and introduced myself. Asked her for a quick word. We stepped aside. I wanted to confirm how long their relationship had been stewing. She said it was all very recent. I passed to the next space which happened to be a cul-de-sac filled with Kapoor's *Memory* (2008), a gigantic rusty blimp or ordnance that obliterated the space in the room, crowded out the space, and I crawled into a tiny pocket under the sculpture, hid myself away from view, was crushed and obliterated, started quietly sobbing.

I asked Paul again for his help. "Grow a dick," he said in a jocular spirit. "Here's a tip for the future: go somewhere in Southern Europe, find a bar, and just go home with someone." A friend said the same thing, more or less, lightly, a young guy ignorant of the odds of a 42-year-old falling pregnant naturally. The very thought of standing in a bar, at 42, going home with a drunken stranger, having unprotected sex, all with a secret and sad agenda—the suggestion filled me with horror.

My youngest sister, who is very wise, could not understand why I was so attached to using Paul's sperm. "It would be a disaster," she said. "It wouldn't be a gift. He'd hold it over you. There's no civilized friendship. Listen to me, it isn't like that."

I gave up, abandoned *our child*. I dropped my heart from its thin slippery sack. Let that go.

I had an appointment with Dr. Rogers at the clinic to discuss freezing my eggs. I couldn't help feeling ashamed to be there on my own and if he scented this shame—which I think he did—he kindly overlooked it. I would do an egg (oocyte) collection just as I would if I were doing a full cycle, only this time, without sperm, instead of immediately using those eggs to create embryos I would put them on ice. The eggs would be "vitrified," snap-frozen. The survival rate for eggs after vitrification was about 60 percent. He let me know no one could say how well the eggs would fertilize after thawing nor could he give a number about the likelihood of a thawed egg resulting in pregnancy. As for the health of children conceived after egg-freezing, well, yes, he advised that knowledge in the field was limited.

We did not talk much about side effects. I recall discussing ovarian hyperstimulation syndrome—a potentially life-threatening condition which involved abnormal swelling and fluid retention. It apparently affected around 1 percent of IVF patients. No doubt a complete nightmare for whoever was unlucky enough to get it. But I didn't blink when the doctor mentioned this risk; if he was cavalier then I was the Commander in Chief of Cavaliers. Freezing my eggs seemed like my only chance to take action, to do something, to break out of my force-frozen stasis, my own icy Ninth Circle of Hell. Crack ice with ice! I knew it was far from ideal but it was better than nothing.

At the front desk I handed the receptionist the new consent form filled in by the doctor. I told her I was freezing my eggs. "Oh." She made a correction on the form, crossed out a couple of treatments and charges, replaced them with two others. I was uneasy with the receptionist determining my treatment and asked that the doctor confirm it.

There is an enormous amount of paperwork involved with IVF. There are underlying consents and then consents along the way for each specific treatment. I had another look at the underlying consents. They very clearly spelled out—among other things—that there was no guarantee of success for any procedure; that assisted reproduction has complications (including ovarian hyperstimulation; pelvic infection; damage to the bladder, bowel or blood vessel at the time of egg collection); and that the doctor managing my care might have a financial interest in the clinic. With those consents I felt the same sense of empowerment, fair bargaining, ability to discuss and negotiate a document, as I did when I signed off blindly on the terms and conditions of the latest Adobe update. Take it or leave it: well, not entirely, I was asked if I would allow my unfertilized eggs to be used for laboratory training. I circled No.

The all-up cost to freeze my eggs was around AU$11,300 (US$11,820)—none of which was covered by public health care.

How did I fund all of this, the IVF, cycle after cycle? A screenplay I wrote under a pseudonym went into production. I spent that windfall—a privileged decision I could afford to make. Once on the phone a friend unwittingly said something hurtful. I was moaning about the high cost of IVF and she said, "I know, my sister had to sell her house to buy her kids." *Buy her kids.*

I went back to the nurses.

I love nurses. I have a nurse fetish, I think I acquired it after my illness in my twenties. It's not acutely sexual, unlike the nurse fetish of a male friend who managed to spark an affair with a nurse while recovering from a heart operation. (No one ever said he had to *buy his life.*) I love nurses because they are kind. I love submitting to their care. At the clinic the nurses played a large role in the IVF treatment. During a cycle they were the point of first and frequent contact. I say "the nurses" because they had their own division: when

I called the nurses, or the nurses called me with a result, I wasn't always sure exactly whom I'd be speaking to—it could have been any nurse from the greater body of nurses. In this way "the nurses" were a kind of timeless ideal, swap out one nurse for another and the nurses would remain untouched in their humble glory. Because I started the process at the city clinic my early visits to the nurses for tests happened at that location, but when it came time to do the egg collection we decided it would be better if I moved to a sister clinic in a suburb closer to my home. The daily monitoring would be easier that way, less travel time. My results would be sent back to the city clinic, which would remain my "operational headquarters." I did have a favorite nurse at the local clinic. Rebecca. Scottish, with pale blond hair, pale skin, soft and pillowy. She was the most adept with the needle. I learned to ask on arrival at reception if she was working that day, as a strong hint I would like to see her. Also, this was awkward, there was a nurse who had twice massacred my arm and by asking after Rebecca I hoped to avoid her. Rebecca was so kind; Gerasima to my Ivana Ilyich. What grace—to take blood from all these women every morning, day in and day out, to know of the great unspoken hope and misery, the high stakes, to greet each patient with a gentle smile and no judgment.

At my orientation session, reorientation session, a city nurse talked me through the three types of needle I'd need to use in the course of the egg collection. She demonstrated on a little patch of fake skin: a square of foam covered in plastic the color of milky tea. I had a few practice jabs myself. Before leaving I was reminded that counseling was available anytime I wanted.

On Day 2 of my period I had my blood tested for FSH, progesterone, and estrogen. That afternoon I got the call from the nurses that my hormone levels were good and that I could start with one injection of 200 IU of Gonal-f in the evening, a moderate dose because this was the first time and the doctor needed to gauge how my body responded. Gonal-f is an artificial hormone, made from recombinant DNA, structurally identical to human follicle stimulating hormone. Scientists tested its efficacy on female rats. Common side effects include headache, ovarian cysts, nausea, upper respiratory tract infections, mastalgia, abdominal pain, diarrhea, vomiting, dizziness, sinus infections, vaginal bleeding, fatigue, back pain, and mood swings. In addition, serious pulmonary conditions have been reported, such as acute respiratory distress syndrome. Rare cases involving blood clots have resulted in death. The basic principle was that by injecting myself with an unnaturally high amount of this hormone I would stimulate my ovaries to overproduce eggs. Usually each month the body naturally releases one mature egg (on rare occasions, two). At age 42, with stimulation, best case was releasing something in the realm of ten to fifteen eggs. The balancing act was to produce as many eggs as possible without causing ovarian hyperstimulation.

The advice was to do injections at around the same time each night so I chose 10 p.m. because that way I wouldn't have to cancel too many evening engagements. Even then, I did have to duck out of dinners early, make excuses. Thankfully, the Gonal-f injection wasn't too bad. Because it didn't involve piercing the vein, taking blood from veins, I convinced myself I could manage it. The delivery mechanism was efficient. I swabbed myself with disinfectant, dialed up the amount of hormone on a pen, unwrapped a needle tip from its packaging and screwed it into the pen, then picked a spot on my belly, about two inches below the belly button, either to the right side or the left. I laid everything out before me as if I were a surgeon about to undertake a major operation. There was a moment when I had to overcome an instinctive aversion to injecting myself, a bit like the moment I face every time I get into the swimming pool. I love to swim, but each immersion requires overcoming an aversion to the affront of cold water. Deep exhale: inject. Hold for ten seconds. Breathe and count. Carefully release. Unscrew needle tip and put in a sharps container. Pack it all away and put back in the fridge, next to the butter and the lettuce. Most times the injection passed without incident. I did jab myself once when careless, also I panicked that I'd screwed the needle tip in too tight and that I'd break the glass vial trying forcefully to unscrew it. When each injection was over I felt a small sense of accomplishment. Done. The methodical experience lent itself to *a sense of purpose.* One part of international travel that I have always enjoyed is making a connecting flight, being alert, following an anonymous fluoro-lit corridor through no-man's-land and thinking of nothing more than getting from A to B: pure and simple. There is comfort in purpose. Part of me wanted to have a child just so I could have an inviolable reason for being. Sweet purpose. Sweet dark purpose, secret of secrets: a child would save my life.

For a two-week period the clinic monitored me closely for effects of the hormone load. This involved almost daily blood tests. After the results came in, usually around midday, I would get a call from the nurses with advice on my next dosage. With every instruction the nurse would say something like "The doctor would like you to do X, Y, Z . . ." so that even if I never saw the doctor I would know he was there, behind the scenes. I had my first trans-vaginal ultrasound on Day 6. The nurse was very kind, applied the goop to her instrument and went about the procedure in a straightforward manner. Still, it was undeniably strange to be lying there, legs spread, feeling something probe around internally, all the while looking at a screen showing a number of dark blobs which—I was told—were my follicles, the sacs of fluid containing my eggs. The nurse took the dimensions of each follicle and measured the thickness of my endometrium. In all, I had nine follicles of a promising size, a potential nine eggs maturing. I felt nine times bloated and nine times labile. I couldn't read the newspaper without crying.

A second needle was introduced to my nightly regime. I would continue with the Gonal-f but add Orgalutran which would stop the eggs from releasing: they had to remain in place for collection. That needle was a little more difficult than the Gonal-f. The needle tip itself was thicker and it required more force, more overcoming, to puncture the skin. I also had a reaction to it: some redness and swelling. Sometimes there was a kind of bubbling under the skin. Quite normal, I was assured. The hormones built up, snow in the night. After another ultrasound and more monitoring a blood test detected a sharp increase in my body's luteinizing hormone, known as the LH surge, an indicator I was naturally readying to ovulate in the next twenty-four to forty-eight hours. My belly was swollen, I was busting to get those eggs out. I was given an exact time to inject Ovidrel, the third and final needle, known as the trigger shot. Press the trigger, release the eggs. It was drilled into me that the timing of the trigger shot was critical; the clinic had coordinated a requisite thirty-six to thirty-eight hour window between the trigger and the time of my scheduled operation. I carried out my instructions with the precision of an astronaut.

In the taxi on the way to the facility—part outpatient surgery, part lab, part clinic—it occurred to me that it would be a terrible time to have a car accident. The building itself—the place where all the precious embryos were stored—was nondescript, fronting a major road. A catastrophist, I also wondered what would happen if the facility burned down: all those dreams would perish.

Surgery is an adventure: I told myself this as I took the elevator to reception. *Curious and curiouser.* I paid money and signed more consents. I spoke first with the administrators; then with the nurses; then with the anesthetist; then with the doctor (faintly comic in his paper shower cap). I tried to meditate during the intervals of waiting. There was a reassuring efficiency to the process: time was of the essence, clearly, but there was no sense of hurry. I gave myself over, submitted to their ministrations. *First, do no harm.* It had been explained to me that even though I had nine follicles on the ultrasound I might not end up with nine eggs. This was because not all follicles contain eggs and it was possible there could be "technical problems" with the doctor's retrieval. Please doctor, have a steady hand. I stripped off my clothes and put on a disposable gown. Laid on the cold trestle table. "I'm going to need your help," said the anesthetist and he asked me to lift my legs into the padded stirrups. A lab scientist or technician read something out for me to confirm. So sci-fi, I couldn't quite believe I was doing it. A cannula went into the top of my hand. And then I was unconscious. When I revived I had a piece of masking tape stuck to my palm with the number six written on it in black felt-tip pen. My teeth would not stop chattering. The number six, what did that mean? A nurse told me six eggs had been collected for freezing. I asked for some Endone to relieve my cramps: made the most of the facility. After a period of observation I was allowed to go home. I called a taxi.

An aside: the day I was instructed to use the Ovidrel trigger I was also given another pen of Gonal-f 900 IU. Each pen cost AU$572 (US$598). The reason for this anomaly was because the treatment is heavily reliant on the results of the morning's blood test and sometimes the body—essentially mysterious—reacts in ways that are not anticipated. When I returned the unopened pen to the clinic the receptionist asked me if I had kept it cold. I told her she shouldn't think about reissuing it. No problem: the pen wasn't reissued, nor was I charged. I got the feeling that $500 was loose change that had slipped behind the sofa.

I didn't ask my sisters or a friend to pick me up from the facility. I wanted to minimize the whole experience, get it over with. I felt foolish. Pathetic. The fact that this had been a spermless dry run with no chance of an embryo was unbearable. On the way back I couldn't have cared less if I died in a car crash. Imagine: the car tumbling off the side of the bridge. How soothing. All the rats came out to play. My anger at Paul was icy cold. Imagine: his car tumbling off the side of the bridge, along with his new family. And midair, struck by a laser beam, totally evaporated. Even my spiteful fantasies were hollow and impotent—that too made me sad. I planned a greeting for the next time I bumped into him—"What makes you think I don't hate you?"

At the same time as I was freezing my eggs I put feelers out about getting some sperm. I asked a dear friend whom I respected a great deal, ten years younger, a single father, living on the far side of the world. He was planning to visit Australia and I hoped that when he was here he could make a donation. It was a flawed plan from the outset because I was unaware the clinic could not turn around a sperm donation in a week, the length of his visit. I'd mistakenly thought the process would be simple: a few papers to sign, the deed itself, and Bob's your father. On the phone I said, "I have a big ask I would have liked to do in person but it's not possible. Would you consider being a sperm donor? No financial responsibility, no custody." Wow: he asked for time to think about it. We spoke again a couple of weeks later. "It's been on my mind every day but I just can't do it. Not for the reason you probably think but because I can't imagine that amazing kid being out there and me not being the father. I couldn't handle knowing you might meet someone and another man would bring up the child. You'd be an amazing mother, it would be an amazing kid, but I can't. I'm so sorry it's not what you want to hear."

Very stupidly, I asked an ex-lover who was married. The idea appealed to him. He wanted to know if he would have to tell his wife. Yes. That fell over.

I was talking to my sister as she was driving down the coast with her husband and two boys. I updated her on the latest sperm rejection. "Just use my hubby's," she said. “You can use it. I’ll ask him.” She asked then and there in the car. “Sure,” he said. “Why not.” It happened so quickly—their tremendous act of kindness.

Because I live by the beach I have quite a few friends who volunteer as lifesavers. They are all strong swimmers who unlike me have mastered their fear of heavy swell and they can go out into the surf in all kinds of weather. One night I was at dinner with three lifesavers and I asked if anyone had ever actually saved a life. Yes, they had: one friend was strolling along an unpatrolled city beach in autumn when she noticed someone face-down in the water. Her first thought was—That’s a weird place to scuba dive. Then as she got closer she realized the person was in trouble. She raced into the water, fully clothed, and dragged the man back to shore. He wasn’t breathing. She did everything right—the mouth-to-mouth and CPR—and when he was taken away in the ambulance he was alive. She didn’t visit him in the hospital, never had any contact with him again. One of those things. The other two lifesavers had paddled out while on patrol to rescue those who were drowning.

My sister’s husband began his visits to the clinic.

He was assessed for eligibility, gave his medical history, went through an overview of the consent forms, did his various blood tests, a urine test. He gave a sperm sample and after it was tested he returned to give more that could go into frozen storage. The known donor sperm workup cost AU$930 (US$966). I never asked him for any details about how he managed ejaculating upwards into a cup. The clock for the quarantine period was set ticking. One thing: we waited for a month to get back the sperm analysis. This was a failure of communication. Things do slip through the cracks. The patient learns to be vigilant.

Once the quarantine period had started the counseling began. My sister and her husband went to the clinic together and talked with a counselor about the legal framework of a donation and the implications for their family. What would they say to their two boys? What if I had a girl, would my sister feel jealous? It was a thorough process. A time was scheduled for the three of us to return together for a second group counseling session, something I dreaded. In our wildest girlhood fantasies about future husbands and babies (our wild-straight fantasies) we never imagined this scenario. In addition, my sister's husband was required to do genetic counseling and undertake a series of genetic tests to identify any chromosomal abnormalities, cystic fibrosis or thalassemia (a disease of the red blood cells). Some results would take three to six weeks to come in. He asked his mother to draw up his family tree, a full family medical history, as required by the clinic. None of us realized the extent of what would be involved when we set out and he dispatched each chore with good grace. We joked about our family topiary.

My sister called with some bad news. She'd been to a BBQ and her father-in-law had made it clear that he was strongly opposed to the sperm donation. "Over my dead body," were the words he used. He worried about his grandchildren. The very concept of IVF did not sit well with him: "I'm sorry but it's not right." She said they were still prepared to go ahead if I really wanted but now it was harder for her husband, who had a close bond with his dad. "Thanks for letting me know," I said. I was tiny. Dearest sister. Who wants to cause a family rift, who wants a child to be born in a storm? I chose not to go ahead and drank the brew of time wasted.

I longed to ask Paul once more for his frozen sperm but knew it would be pointless. *Our child* clung to me like a ghost.

One morning I woke up and noticed a tiny black mark on my palm, like a nascent melanoma. Maybe a blood blister. I waited to see if it would sink away but after a week it hadn't changed. Then it started to grow bigger, almost imperceptibly, the way the body usually changes. I tried scratching if off but that didn't work. Something else: it was hard, not as soft as a mole. I hoped it would go away. Instead it kept growing, it reached the size of a small coin and then it started to thicken, protrude. It took the shape of a spike or a blade, there in the hollow of my palm. I had to walk around with my hand curled into a fist in order to hide it. Late one night, when I couldn't sleep, I turned on my side and began pounding the bed, the empty space where my husband used to lie. I had grown my knife, now I was compelled to use it. I was sure that was the only way to get it out of my hand. My father used to complain that my mother hit him in his sleep. Back then I'd never understood it.

A prince came to my rescue. I walked up to his castle, knocked on the door. We'd had a dalliance some twenty-odd years earlier and since then had kept in touch. I told him of my predicament. In turn, he grilled me about why I wanted a child. He wanted to know the state of my finances. He reminded me that having a child wasn't all fun and games, wasn't easy. "Take your niece home for two weeks or two months, see how you like it. Your whole life will change." He said he'd think it over—and soon came back saying yes, I deserved a chance, he'd help me. *Darling man!* The good news was that he already had frozen sperm in storage, at another clinic, so hopefully I wouldn't have to wait out the quarantine period. His one condition: he wanted our arrangement to be strictly confidential—for the first three years of the child's life. I wouldn't be able to tell anyone he was the donor. I agreed. We drafted a legal document that extensively outlined the expectations of the Mother and the Donor, pre- and post-conception. Basically it said he would have no financial responsibility, no custody: he would not be the legal parent. I think we did discuss trying to get pregnant the good old-fashioned way—sleeping together—but under the law that would mean he would have unwanted responsibilities. We took a very straight, strict approach. *Strait is the gate.* I felt hopeful and grateful when I signed on as the Mother.

The Mother. I allowed myself some small leeway to identify as a mother, to peek through the door. Both my sisters had set an example. I am enchanted by my nieces and nephews. For many of my nephews' early years I was living overseas and didn't spend that much time with them. My nieces were born when I was 41 and 44. Their mother was intimately aware of my difficult circumstances. I had a choice: I could distance myself from her pregnancies in order to spare myself pain, or I could embrace them. Today I am so glad that I did not hide away, cut myself off, that I chose a path that at times was excruciating, bittersweet. There were nights when I was babysitting and would cry when checking on the sleeping child, there were days when I couldn't stand another minute in the swarming playground. Birthday parties remain a bridge too far. In spending time with the baby girls a new kind of love was revealed to me, one that emanated directly from the chest, something uncomplicated and all-forgiving. It was different in tenor to the great love I'd had for my husband—which also emanated directly from the chest but which, I am not proud to say, proved more complicated, less forgiving. This new way of loving was something gentle and constant. A plain good thing.

PROSECUTOR: Why did you persist in wanting to be a mother?
DEFENSE: I refer you to Exhibit A. Conversation with Elsie, age 2.

—Let's play doctors and mices! Doctors and mices!
—OK, what's that?
—You say, "A mouse is coming!"
—A mouse is coming!

I make my hand into a mouse, creep it close to her, then run the mouse-hand under her arms, begin to tickle. Soon the mouse-hand bounces up and down on her tummy.

—I'm not a trampoline! I'm not a trampoline! I'm not a trampoline! I'm a person!
—Oh, OK.
—Do it on your nose!

The mouse-hand bounces up and down on my nose.

—Your nose is a trampoline!

Mother's Day was a punch in the gut.

I had a friend also doing IVF but in Europe, who was much more sanguine. She said her whole family was in good health, she had amazing friends, she loved her work, she lived in a wonderful city, and after much heartbreak she now spent every day alongside her beloved new husband. "Too much for one person, don't you think?" They were seriously considering adoption. Perhaps if I'd had that option—adoption—I would have been less fervent. In a country with extremely tight adoption laws I reckoned my chance of adopting at approximately zero. Anyway, selfishly, at the outset I wasn't that keen on adoption.

And now it was my donor's turn to begin his visits to the clinic. He had an appointment with the doctor; an appointment alone with the counselor; and we did a joint counseling session together. There were consents to consider. (A donor always owned his sperm and could withdraw his consent at any time.) The quarantine had to be verified and the blood work reviewed so that it met all the standards of my clinic. His genetic screening also had to be reviewed. It turned out that since we'd both done our initial screening for cystic fibrosis a new test that covered a greater spectrum of mutations had become available and we needed to do that. I also redid my AMH and a lot of other things. Because of my donor's family history the genetic counselor advised we needed to consider a range of potential chromosomal problems. There was a test that could be done at a hospital lab on the other side of town. I hesitated to overburden my donor, fearful he too might change his mind, so I decided I would be the one to take the test. If the results proved negative—which I expected—then the genetic counselor had advised I could put it out of my mind. Both parents needed to have the mutation for there to be a risk of passing it on to the child. Another thing had changed since my donor first froze his sperm. The law now required that at birth all donors be registered so that a child conceived with donor sperm could one day trace the father. He was happy with that.

The straws of sperm were shipped from one clinic to another. One precious straw was tested for the sperm's motility and possible deformations. Under the microscope everything was swimming. When it was already too late I was ready to go.

After consulting with the doctor I chose to proceed with an IUI, intrauterine insemination, at a cost of AU$2,040 (US$1,832) of which around $670 (US$602) would be reimbursed by Medicare. I would do it with a nudge of Gonal-f, 75 IU, to boost my chances. On Day 9 the clinic would start monitoring me for my LH surge. I also had an ultrasound. It was similar to using a turkey baster at home (although I had heard the best way wasn't a turkey baster but a plastic syringe acquired at any local pharmacy). Why did I involve the clinic, why not try at home? Well, I wanted the donor's sperm to have cleared the HIV risk, and—more than that—I wasn't sure he would have been comfortable making home deliveries. And why not go straight to IVF? My thinking was that my eggs had never had a chance: the problem had been my husband's lack of sperm. I hoped that if my egg was exposed to healthy sperm then I wouldn't need to undertake the more invasive, and expensive, IVF.

On the appointed day of ovulation I arrived at the facility. A nurse—there was no doctor involved—tried to insert a fine plastic tube into my cervix but after a good ten minutes of prodding, failing, she gave up, apologized and left the room to find another nurse. *Alone, alone.* The second nurse had better luck. The thawed sperm—which had also been rinsed and concentrated—was injected directly into my uterus. It was uncomfortable, like having a bad period cramp. I asked if I could keep lying down for fifteen minutes. Quietly excited, I tried to visualize conception, the sperm and the egg. I placed my hands on my belly and sent loving energy to the womb. My doctor had said I could stand on my head and meditate if I wanted but that kind of thing wouldn't make any difference. I paid no heed. After I left, in a lane off the main road, I found a paperbark tree and peeled away some bark, placed it under my T-shirt, gently rubbed my skin in a circular motion. Absurd—but who cares. It was soothing. I believe in ceremony. Anything to counter the unnatural situation.

My friend in New York paid a surrogate. "She lives in a beautiful place, interstate, so much nature. The whole thing felt really natural." Nature. Natural. She continued to repeat the word "natural" like a nervous tic or mantra.

The day after the procedure I called my sister in an embarrassed small panic. I'd absentmindedly eaten some sushi, which was a no-no according to one of the books I'd read, *What to Eat When You're Expecting.* "Oh my god, you're fine," she said. "You can snort heroin for breakfast at this stage and you'll be fine. Don't be insane. It's not going to be like this the whole time, is it?"

Good morning, darling. Every day I greeted my belly as if an embryo had implanted. Disregarding the odds of success I directed a loving monologue to what I hoped existed. I'd long harboured a platonic crush on my donor, considering him a trusted battle-worn compadre, and I believed the child of our friendship was also meant-to-be. (Did I still carry grief for the lost *our child*? Yes, of course I did.) During that first two-week wait I had a heightened awareness of my whole body. Rarely did I ever stop to consider how my body was functioning, what my cells were doing. Typically I completely ignored the subtle movements that go on all the time: the inflating, deflating lung; the inch of chyme through the intestine; the tremors of the liver and the kidneys. Not that I actually felt these things, but I pictured them, sensed them. What is that way of knowing? Out on the street I noticed that all the babies, toddlers, and pregnant women had cloned themselves so now they were everywhere. I smiled at young mothers. I was soft and optimistic, the holder of a wonderful secret. It's easy to do anything once.

Blood. Bloody hell. Hopes raised, hopes dashed. But I wasn't devastated: no need to take a fall straight out of the blocks. My mother was right when she said "It would have been an absolute miracle." I opted to immediately do a second IUI, again supported with nightly injections of Gonal-f. It was impossible to gauge the quality of my eggs with only one try. I was monitored regularly—but not daily—and when the nurse called me with my scheduled time for the procedure I queried if the time wasn't too late, if it were possible the LH surge could have begun on the day before when I wasn't tested, if too many hours could have passed between an undetected surge and the procedure. She referred me to the doctor. He said: "I've seen the numbers a thousand times. This is how we do it. You have to trust me." I asked him to quickly explain how the time window worked. "If you don't trust me," he replied, "we can cancel."

The second IUI failed. As a next step Dr. Rogers recommended I use my frozen eggs and also do a fresh cycle at the same time. I took that to mean I'd do a new cycle, collect a new batch of fresh eggs, inseminate them, and at the same time, thaw the frozen eggs, inseminate them too.

—Why not just use the frozen?
—You get more with both.
—I've already got five frozen so why do I need more?
—Up to you.
—Is there a difference between fresh and frozen?
—There are no second-class children.
—I mean, is one more viable than the other?
—Not much difference.
—OK, I'll just do frozen.
—Whatever you want. That's reasonable.

Up to you. Pick your own misadventure.

Coffee. At the orientation the dietary advice I received from the clinic was to moderate my coffee and alcohol intake and take folic acid, 500 mcg daily. I asked what was "moderate" and was told one cup a day would be fine. A million websites and bulletin boards advised no coffee. They also advised countless other things. Stay alkaline. Wear a lead-lined apron on airplanes. Avoid bananas. I decided to cut out coffee completely. After three months of IVF failure I reverted back to one cup a day. I trawled the Internet and found the study about caffeine . . . it concluded that five cups a day was to be discouraged. Sometimes I felt guilty when I had my morning coffee: what if this coffee was the one thing between me and pregnancy? Most times I thought if one coffee a day kills my chance that dear embryo-darling wasn't strong enough to last the nine months anyway. I oscillated between guilt and pragmatism, and that movement, that kinetic energy, helped drive the little engine of endurance.

I saw Paul at the pool. *Vampire! Monster!* I swam as if I were drowning, thrashing the water, wild-armed, wrenching my head from side to side. I moved fast. No chance to ruminate. At the end of each lap I paused to catch my breath. Exhausted.

The month after the second failed IUI I readied for a frozen egg cycle at an out-of-pocket cost of AU$2,705 (US$2,597). Again I was monitored closely so that we could time the transfer of the embryo to be in sync with my natural cycle. The frozen eggs would be thawed and artificially inseminated the day I naturally ovulated. I was told that three out of five eggs had survived the thaw and they had been injected with sperm selected under digital high-magnification by a scientist, a procedure called intracytoplasmic sperm injection or ICSI. Actually I always did ICSI—the doctors never recommended straight IVF, which is where the sperm fight it out in the Petri dish en route to the egg. ICSI cost an additional $730 (US$701) which in the scheme of things felt nominal (how quickly the scales transmogrify). Later I read a study that questioned why so many doctors always recommended ICSI, speculating there may be some benefit to a stronger, fitter sperm fighting its way to the egg in the Petri dish, just as it did under the auspices of Mother Nature. Overnight one embryo showed development—but it was atypical. "It contains three pieces of genetic information." Three pieces of genetic information! The nurse told me that it couldn't be transferred. My sister and I joked about dirty pipettes but in fact my egg had divided abnormally and carried an extra set of chromosomes. The nurse had further bad news: my remaining two embryos had shown no development. They would be kept another night and checked in the morning to see if there were any changes: I was warned this was unlikely but not impossible. I had been out on a boat that day, up and down, up and down, rolling on the heavy swell, and come evening I had full-blown vertigo. If I dipped my chin an inch to look at a screen I felt as if I were about to pitch face-first off a cliff. The next morning, in my vertiginous state, I got the polite, carefully delivered news that there were no signs of improvement. All five embryos were to be "discarded." All five—gone, tossed away, *discarded*. For a long moment I was silent and then I quietly asked the lab assistant, "You definitely destroy them?" It troubled me how invisible everything was: how would I know what they really did with my embryos? Who monitored the checks and balances? Scenarios for horror movies made themselves known. Evil lab assistant sells embryos on baby black market; evil doctor fertilizes eggs with own sperm to create own private colony of children; evil research director conducts clandestine experiments to grow babies full-term ex-uterus . . . As it happened, in all my five subsequent egg collections I had a much better success rate with embryo development, always ending up with something that could be transferred.

I was having trouble sleeping so in the middle of the night I walked down to the playground at the end of my street. All the ghost-children were at play. There were little boys crawling over webs of rope, little girls kicking up their heels on the swings. They sang and squabbled and thrilled at making footprints in the dirt. I told a girl I loved her outfit. "It's not an outfit!" she said. "It's a tiger suit!" A black-haired boy sat beside me and whispered in my ear, "Change doctors."

I went back to the same clinic website and found a new doctor, to be known as Dr. Nell. My GP wrote a referral. No one at the clinic asked any awkward questions as to why I was switching. On the wall of Dr. Nell's office was a noticeboard pinned with thank-you cards and baby photos. Her manner was kind and thoughtful. We discussed my options for the next cycle. I'd do a new egg collection. She raised some "optional extras" that were available as part of the service. The first was a chromosomal test that could be done on the embryo that would cost an additional AU$3,670 (US$3,347). It was especially helpful, she said, for women who'd had recurring miscarriages. That test needed to be booked months in advance so I didn't opt for it. For $265 (US$242) I was also offered "assisted hatching," whereby a lab technician would use a laser to thin the outer shell of the embryo, making it easier—supposedly—for the embryo to "hatch out" prior to implantation. Older women, I was told, have a harder "outer shell." The procedure carried a small risk of penetrating the shell and damaging the embryo. And on top of that—if I wanted—I could try "embryo glue" for $150 (US$137); this was also supposed to aid implantation. I asked her whether there was evidence for increased chances of success with the assisted hatching and the embryo glue. *They apply pigeons, to draw the vapors from the head.* She said there was no clear evidence but that if I went ahead I could say I'd done all I could. "What would you do if you were in my shoes?" I asked. She said, "It's up to you." This time I didn't use the glue but I did in subsequent cycles. The cost ended up being $9,675 (US$8,824) plus anesthetist and outpatient surgery fees on top.

Medicare reimbursed just under $5,200 (US$4,742). I had the dread feeling that I was voluntarily participating in "cutting-edge" medicine, that I was a part of some greater experiment, a credulous and desperate older woman, and the only thing that made me think these dread thoughts might be mere anxiety, that actually I was the lucky beneficiary of years of advanced medical research, was the calm and caring manner of my doctor, who on a personal level did seem sincere in her desire to help me fall pregnant, just as she had helped all the women who had sent her those colorful cards pinned to her wall.

One of the last conversations I had with Dr. Nell was along the following lines:

—Is there anything we would do differently next cycle?
—No.
—If you were a crazy experimentalist and I were a willing research participant, what would you suggest?
—We could try testosterone treatment for three weeks before the cycle.
—Testosterone? What's that for?

—It helps egg quality.

—How come I'm only hearing about it now?

—There have been three studies in the past year.

—Is testosterone something the clinic offers their patients?

—We decide patient by patient. I know you like to see the evidence so I didn't think you'd want the testosterone. There's not enough evidence yet.

—Well, what else is there?

—Growth hormone—but I wouldn't offer you that because it does have links to cancer.

—So we wouldn't do anything different?

—No.

On Day 1 of my next period I called the nurses. I was told to come in that morning for a blood test. On other occasions I'd done my initial bloods on Day 2 and so I asked if there was a reason why I needed to come in on Day 1. The nurse said, "We can always go forward but we can't go back." That afternoon I received a call.

—Bad news, I'm afraid. Doctor has looked at the results and wants to cancel the cycle. High FSH.

—That's unusual, that hasn't happened before.

—It hasn't been looked at before.

—Yes it has, I did a frozen cycle. How high was my FSH?

—13.

—And how high was it when I did the frozen cycle? Please check the file.

—11.

—Why did we take the bloods on Day 1? Maybe the FSH will go down by Day 2. Is it OK if I come in and test again on Day 2?

—Yes, come in.

My Day 2 FSH result dropped to 11.7. The doctor—not Dr. Nell but another doctor who was covering for her while she was away—decided the level was still too high and the cycle had to be canceled. When I asked the nurse about why my FSH might have been high she said, simply, "It's cyclical, doctor said wait until next month." When I got off the phone I cried. I had a great fear that I was too old, that my FSH would remain too high. The process was forever throwing up new ways to be disappointed that I hadn't even dreamt existed. The constant uncertainty took a toll.

In expectation of proceeding with the cycle I'd canceled a work trip. There were so many opportunities I turned down in the course of my treatment.

One afternoon I struck up a conversation with a mendacious cab driver. He said, "I have seven sons, age 2 to 14. I'm 74. My wife is 62. She had the first four compulsory and then three voluntary because she wanted a girl. Yes, she was 60! I can drive you to my place and show you her passport! I drive this cab and do all the cooking and cleaning. I sleep four hours. I feel young. To be honest, it's not her I love, it's the kids."

November 2013. I felt a small sense of pride when the nurse told me this month's levels were good—FSH down to 7.7, estrogen 202—as if somehow I had worked hard to deserve this merit. *This is the start of an amazing journey.* I blazed with hope. I was injecting 300 IU of Gonal-f each night. My breasts became extremely sensitive. Once again I was bloated and labile. When I put my travel card into the ticket machine on the bus I felt as if I were inserting my own fingers. I cut everything out—coffee, dairy, sugar, alcohol (that was hard). Each day I drank an alkalizer juice from the health food store. I kept up my iodine-folate and multivitamin and added fish oil. All the small rituals. After my scan—which looked promising—the kind nurse said, "Hope you get some in the freezer." That was my wish: to do a fresh transfer with one embryo and have others "left over" to freeze. Dr. Nell was away again on the day of my egg collection so it fell to a new doctor I'd never seen before to explain that in fact I wouldn't be able to do a fresh transfer that month, as planned. My last blood test had shown an unexpectedly high level of progesterone, a hormone produced by the ovary that plays a decisive factor in maintaining pregnancies.

—Your progesterone is at 6 so we can't do a fresh transfer.

—Sorry, what does that mean?

—Your body has started producing progesterone before ovulating. There's nothing we could have done about it. It means the lining of your uterus will be out of sync with implantation. It could implant, it's not impossible, but the window isn't optimum. I don't want you to look back and say "Why did we waste this embryo?"

—What's the cut-off for progesterone?

—5. And yours was 6, it wasn't 5.1 or 5.2. Some clinics in the U.S. freeze all embryos and don't do fresh transfers.

—So you're giving me strong advice? Nothing wishy-washy?

—I can only advise you. It's up to you to do what you want.

—But I have no medical experience.

—Well, that's my advice. Check with Dr. Nell when she's back on Monday. You can take the pessaries until then, there's no harm in that.

Eleven eggs were collected, of which seven were mature. These mature eggs were injected with sperm. Overnight, four of the seven embryos showed signs of developing. By Day 3 only one embryo was going strong, with another two looking borderline. The lab assistants—always women—updated me on the process of attrition. I had to steel my nerves each time they called. By Day 5 I was left with one Grade A blastocyst—which quality-wise was the best outcome possible. The clinic had a complex system for grading embryos depending on the progression of cell division: a blastocyst was a Day 5 embryo that had developed a distinctive shape with an inner cell mass clearly identifiable within its fluid-filled cavity. A blastocyst had the best chance of resulting in a pregnancy. That said, embryos *less developed* than a blastocyst had also been known to be viable so there was—as ever—a wide spectrum of hope.

Dr. Nell had returned to her office and I asked her again what she would do if she were in my shoes: a fresh or frozen transfer? This time she answered unequivocally, "If it were me I'd definitely freeze."

I was disoriented by the numbers, the odds, as if I were playing a game in which I didn't know the rules, "Kindly Kafka."

—When you say my progesterone was 6 what does that mean? Was it 6 out of 10 or 6 out of 100?
—It's not out of anything. It's a number and our cut-off is 5.
—Is it true fresh transfers are better than frozen transfers?
—Some clinics in Spain only ever do frozen transfers.
—But what if the defrost doesn't work? I only have one embryo.

—The rate is 90 percent for a successful embryo defrost. Weighing it all up, my advice is to freeze.

The horror, the horror: a 10 percent chance it won't defrost.

—All right, let's freeze.

An uncharitable thought . . . IVF seemed to be a great deal about levels and cut-offs. If number X, then do Y. I wondered if it was the medical equivalent of conveyancing in the legal world, which is to say, largely formulaic, a matter of following protocol.

The lab was closed for Christmas break and also undergoing renovations so I had to wait until January to do my transfer. A friend had been following my travails, she herself was a veteran of IVF, now a blessedly happy and exhausted mother. I told her it was ridiculous but I was sad to think of my darling little embryo spending Christmas all alone in a freezing cold tank of liquid nitrogen. "It won't be alone," she said. "Our siblings are there too." We are all lunatics. She had gone through the same clinic and was successful when she gave up trying with her own eggs and moved to using her husband's sperm with a donor egg from a young woman in her twenties, one of her close friends. That child is adorable. Her view is that the science of IVF is as astonishing as the science that put a man on the moon. Her gratitude to her doctor is enormous. In her eyes he is like a pioneer or astronaut. He is working at the forefront of miracle and wonder.

I bought my nephews a crazy number of presents for Christmas.

One day I was babysitting and after I'd nagged the boys to put away their LEGO the youngest commented, "You don't have kids so you don't know how we work."

By Day 31 I still hadn't got my period. Never before in my life had this happened to me. I worried that because I'd done yoga in a heated room for a week I might have inadvertently messed things up; I worried that something dire had happened when I'd been slammed in my belly, bang on my right ovary, while playing tennis; I worried, I worried. I had a blood test on Day 33, which also happened to be my 44th birthday. "Happy Birthday," said the nurse as she read out my birthdate. We laughed. She thought it a pity I had to come in that day; I told her it was auspicious. When I left the clinic I noticed a man, a grandfather, leading a toddler across the street. Toddling. I felt a flush of heartwarmth at the sight of that little girl. Could she be enough for me? Did I need to place my own child at the center of the world? Was it enough that other beautiful children existed? If I could make the revolutionary shift from *I* to *We*, from *I* to *This*, perhaps that would be possible.

At last my transfer was scheduled. I woke at 6 a.m. and took a cab to an acupuncture clinic in the city that a friend had recommended. It was a public holiday, ghostly, no one else was around. Bend the rules of nature, bend the rules of time. The acupuncturist had kindly made a special trip to meet me. I liked her because she called me "darling." I was there because I'd heard that acupuncture on the day of transfer could aid implantation, *potentially* aid implantation—the evidence itself was limited. Half an hour of lying on the table was about all I could take. When the session was finished I took a second cab from the city to the facility and considered the cab driver's Hare Krishna music a good omen. At reception I noticed Paul's name was typed on the consent form as my next of kin so I drew a line through that, pressed down hard with the pen. I was directed to an airlocked changing room, known as the "Clean Room." I felt like Charlie when he first enters the chocolate factory with Willy Wonka, wide-eyed. I removed half of my clothing and put on a hair cap, overshoes, and a blue papery gown. I then pressed a button to release the airlock and passed through to the pristine all-white surgery. A lab adjoined the surgery. I took a seat on what looked like a dentist's chair, spread my legs. There was a lot of identity checking and I had to repeat my name and birthdate in a loud voice because it was all being recorded. The doctor and the lab technician also had to loudly confirm details, which I guessed was part of the protocol for avoiding an embryo mix-up. On Dr. Nell's instruction I held the ultrasound wand over my belly, revealing my inner moonscape on a small screen. There was another screen perched high in the corner of the room that relayed from the lab an image of my embryo, greatly magnified. "It looks good," said the doctor. "It looks just like the one in the book, doesn't it?" Since I didn't remember the images in the info booklet I didn't answer. "Yes," she said loudly, "it looks like the one in the book." The lab technician disappeared the embryo into a fine bendy plastic catheter. She brought this tube to Dr. Nell, who tried to insert it into my cervix, but she had trouble and the lab technician was sent to find a stiffer tube. I know now that the more difficult the actual physical transfer the worse it is for the fragile embryo. On the moonscape screen I saw a minuscule white speck being released from the tube onto my doughnut-shaped uterus. I asked if I was OK to fly, do yoga, go swimming. Yes to all three, with the proviso I don't overheat. "And you can go to the toilet now, it won't fall out." I returned to the acupuncture clinic for a half-hour session of deep relaxation. Afterwards I walked over to the art gallery and saw an exhibition of exquisite Korean ceramics, *Soul of Simplicity.* As I was leaving I spied the bus up ahead and made a run for it. I felt a twinge in my belly. Oh no, what have I done! I'm an idiot! You idiot! Quietly now: you idiot.

I began to wait. "What are my odds—of being pregnant?" was another question I'd asked Dr. Nell on the day of the transfer. Her reply: A Day 5 blastocyst has about a 40 percent chance. *How wonderful, 40 percent!* That night I felt extremely sensual, writhed like a snake, embodied metamorphosis, and avoided pleasuring myself because I feared contractions could disrupt things. The next morning I had a tiny amount of brown spotting which I'd read was an indicator of implantation. Oh the delight. And then, immediately, tamp down delight. Wait. Wait and see. My friend who subscribed to Chinese medicine strongly advised I cut out cold swims. "The little bean needs a warm nest." So I did that. I was taking progesterone pessaries morning and night and my breasts swelled, grew sensitive. I hoped and believed I was pregnant. On Day 27 I noticed the slightest discoloration in my urine: a hint of blood. And I collapsed. Howled. Wept. Even though there was no full bleed I sensed my period was imminent. Down, down, down the rathole. The air there was thick and dull. My skin flushed, goose-pimpled. My eyes stang red-raw. My jaw clamped tight. I felt utterly bereft. Alone, alone. You have fucked up your life. The rats of the world scuttled and gnawed. I found it impossible to leave the house.

To make myself feel better I broke a vow and Googled my ex-husband. (A frightening thought: am I a brilliant masochist?) There he was—happy, smiling. In a Facebook photo his new partner sat on the sidelines watching him play cricket. Resentment is a curse. Repulsive: like putting on a soiled garment. Parading around in it.

This didn't happen: I went to a Goddess Weekend where we worked on our inner Ancient Greek. We sharpened our swords and swore revenge. We hacked our way through grief.

All time was measured according to my menstrual cycle. "January" meant nothing to me. Days closest to my "due date" weighed heaviest. By Day 29 I still hadn't had a full bleed. In the morning I did a blood test and then went to spend the day with my sister. She was eight months or so pregnant. We had lunch at an inner-city café that was popular with young families because of its mock-farm design: wooden pens with some real chickens and a well-fed pig. Little Elsie pointed to a rooster on a weather vane and said "Sky Chicken!" I was overwhelmed—by all the children, the Yummy Mummies, by Café Potemkin. Later we watched *The Wizard of Oz* while I gave my sister a foot massage. My phone rang: it was the nurses calling. From the measured tone of voice I could instantly tell the pregnancy test had been negative—as expected. "You can begin another antagonist cycle now if you want to." When I spoke to the doctor she was gently reassuring: it was good that I had responded well to the egg collection; often it took people two or three tries for chromosomal reasons. "Sometimes an embryo won't implant because of the chromosomes and there's nothing we can do about that." My sister consoled me. I tried to be brave because I didn't want to pollute her.

I went to a dance class. A kind of free-form hippie dance class. A woman in face paint smudged me with burning sage at the door. It felt so good to reconnect with my body. During the night I had an orgasm in my sleep. Throughout my treatment I didn't have sex, which made for the longest period of sexual inactivity I'd ever known. Injecting needles each night at 10 p.m. was unsexy; being bloated and hormonally loaded was unsexy; the white goop of progesterone pessaries during the two-week wait was unsexy; explaining I was doing IVF by myself was unsexy; *I* was unsexy. And recalibrating my fine chemical equilibrium was unnerving. Why invite a bull into the china shop? I'd even say a part of me didn't want to bodily introduce any sperm other than my donor's. Foolish. Minimizing. While doing IVF I allowed the world to become a smaller place.

Ways of having approximate sex: feel the heat of a stranger on public transport during peak hour; finger the downy peaches in the fruit store; call out "Coming!" to the man who brings home delivery to the door.

The baby was born. I attended the birth. Everyone cried with joy. I held the tiny newborn in my arms and smelled her.

How to be an object of pity? My sister has a great answer to this one. "Most people think only about themselves, they don't really care." Other people's pity is flimsy. Harmless. If it even exists, it passes. Other people's compassion is a boon. So it's self-pity that's the killer.

When I went to the counselor at the clinic she drew me a picture. "This is the grief," she said, marking the page with an elongated black hole. "The divorce grief, the infertility grief." She explained that when we were triggered by an event—it could be anything—we returned to the grief. She marked a dot near the black hole and drew a loop between them. She drew lots of dots, lots of small concentric loops. "And then, over time, we find we have fewer triggers." She marked a dot at a greater distance from the black hole, drew a bigger loop. More dots, four bigger loops containing all the other loops.

"See—it's a butterfly." I just nodded. I wanted to take a pin and stick it between my eyes. *Pinned and wriggling on the wall.*

February 2014. Eight eggs were harvested on my third collection. Five of those were mature and were injected with sperm. The lab assistants called on schedule with their morbid countdown. *Please, please develop. You can do it!* I was an embryo cheerleader. I filled those Petri dishes with love. On Day 5, the morning of my transfer, I learned that this time I only had a morula to transfer, not a blastocyst. I'd never heard of a morula before—essentially it is an embryo less developed than a blastocyst but still worth transferring. When I asked the doctor about the difference she said that the pregnancy rate for a morula was 25 percent compared to 40 percent for a blastocyst. My heart fell. Whatever eyes-wide wonder I'd had when first doing a transfer had dissipated and now Charlie's chocolate factory was a factory plain and simple. Efficacious. I didn't enjoy my acupuncture—all those pinpricks—and wondered whether it was worth pursuing. I still had hope the transfer would be successful, I still conducted my inner conversations with the embryo, but my hope wasn't as intense as it had been before. I slept a lot. Snow fell in the night. I paid visits to my sister and the new baby. One day I was wearing a wraparound dress that she said looked handy for breastfeeding so we did a costume change. She lent me a loose blue dress she had worn up until the birth. "If I wear this dress," I joked, "maybe it will rub off and I'll get pregnant." I waited and waited. Come Day 28 there was no sign of bleeding. That shy little hope grew and grew. How kind the nurse was when she took my blood. I held my breath all day waiting for the call. "I'm sorry, it's negative." I told the nurse I was too wrung out to go straight into another cycle. Wept on the floor.

I had my annual conversation with a woman (mother of two) who was once a close friend. "What's next for you? Forget about babies," said the friend. "The baby boat has sailed." *Bitch*: I hadn't breathed a word to her about my treatment. *Wait and see.*

Now I don't care but for a long time I was circumspect about telling people I was doing IVF. Professionally, while there was still a chance I could become pregnant, it wasn't wise. With friends I was careful about who I told. I didn't want to tell my friend with breast cancer because she had enough on her plate; I didn't want to tell my friends who were new mothers and obsessed with their babies; I didn't want to tell friends who either were at ease not being mothers or those who found themselves childless in circumstances similar to mine; nor did I want to tell my friend who had remained close to my ex-husband. I didn't want to tell people because I thought that unless they were involved in that world themselves they wouldn't want to listen. Or they would only half listen and so diminish my experience. Or they would ask questions that required explanations too complex for conversation. Or they would offer advice based on hearsay and a general theory of positivity. Or I would make them uncomfortable because of my proximity to the abyss. *Hush, keep your voice down, don't mention it by name.*

The following month was a respite. Thank all the gods. I jumped on a plane to Bali and for ten days worked on a commissioned script from a villa overlooking the Sayan Ridge in Ubud. The place was lush, verdant, abundantly fertile. Dense and green. I counted six layered storeys of green from my terrace. Vertical green. Ten thousand insects. I luxuriated in having someone bring me breakfast each morning. I did yoga and had massages: unashamed, a walking convalescent. Eat, Pray, Love—or "Eat, Pay, Leave," as the locals say—who cares. It was good. It helped. I'd do it again in a heartbeat.

On resuming treatment I noticed that the white cockatoos who habitually roosted on a nearby roof antenna had fallen silent. It drove me crazy that Paul had turned his back and walked off into the so-called sunset while I was left with my pathetic hormone injections. Callous lotus-eater! Faux Buddhist! Fake feminist! Hey Orpheus, turn around! The rats had a field day. I heard myself referring to "my infertility" when talking to my sister. A slip of the tongue. I'd never applied the term to myself before—I wasn't infertile, I was "trying to get pregnant." To be infertile sounded like something already decided, finalized, irreversible. I had to drag myself back to the nurses. Dread intermingled with hope this time round. I wasn't sure I could withstand another failure. The test of IVF, I came to realize, is to do with both intensity and duration. IVF is durational in the same way a lot of people can sit at a table and stare at a stranger for ten minutes but very few can do it for 700-plus hours. One day after I'd left the clinic I needed to do some shopping and had my carry bag of drugs with me. Those telltale nylon bags, just big enough for a cold pack: all women doing IVF could spot them a mile away. I bought a dozen eggs. Egg kit, eggs in hand: the moment was absurd. I was slipping. Rally! "You are Team Captain," I told myself. "Keep it together. It isn't what happens to a person but how they respond that counts. There is hope. It's not over yet. You are Team Captain. Team Captain." In the evening, after my needle, I practiced a visualization exercise, partially inspired by an engraved medical illustration I'd bought after my lung operation. It's a page cut from a nineteenth-century medical book depicting a bust-sized portrait of a woman, alive, well, fully clothed, her head in three-quarter profile, whose chest is completely open, revealing her lungs and other internal workings. Gruesome and elegant. And hopelessly outmoded by today's medical knowledge. So I pictured my own internal belly workings and saw follicles growing, sprouting out of my ovaries, each follicle a point of light. *Lush, verdant, abundantly fertile.*

And something else about that nineteenth-century engraving: as I was doing IVF it felt like medical science was moving at such a fast pace that whatever the treatment I was being prescribed it was already on the verge of being surpassed. This made for a substrata anxiety about "keeping up with the latest."

When I was in Bali a friend—successful in her treatment—had sworn by DHEA. I'd written to my doctor saying that a non-medical friend had recommended something called DHEA as a possible fertility treatment. What was it and did she think it suitable for me at this stage? The doctor replied that DHEA (dehydroepiandrosterone) was a weak male hormone that can be taken as a tablet three times a day. She said there had been a lot of work looking at DHEA as a way of improving egg quality and ovarian response to stimulation but the studies on the whole showed no improvement and as such there didn't appear to be much benefit in taking it. Still, if I wanted to go ahead she would write me a prescription. Another quandary. I declined.

If anyone says they chose not to have children because the world is already overpopulated, because the world doesn't need any more children, I don't buy it. I also didn't buy it when my friend who has six children said the country needed more children because "otherwise who is going to pay for our retirement?" If a decision really is made, it's telescopically micro, not macro. For instance, I did believe a different friend who said he'd never wanted to have a child because he thought it unfair—unkind—to inflict consciousness on another being.

One mother said to me, "I don't know how you can choose to be pregnant. Our kids weren't planned. I wouldn't have had the courage." My response: "With IVF—you have to choose."

The titanium hook: I only need one and it could be the next one.

I weighed myself down with more hormones. The scan showed nine large follicles. And a blood test revealed that once again my progesterone was high and the possibility of a fresh transfer was thrown in doubt. "I can only advise what I'd do myself," said the doctor. "If you say you want to go ahead I'll still treat you." I chose to wait for a frozen transfer, as I'd done before. The run sheet: seven eggs were collected of which six were mature. Only three fertilized overnight. And by Day 3 of the countdown all three embryos were still going strong, which raised the exciting prospect that for the first time I might be lucky enough to get more than one embryo worthy of being transferred. How eager I was to fan the flame of hope. More than one viable embryo! Blessed bounty! I remember I received the good news when I ducked out of an actors' workshop that I was auditing. Earlier in the day the acting coach—a man—had stopped a 20-something actress midway through her scene. "I can't hear you! Speak up! As a woman you can have a voice, you're not a child or a girl! Listen to this—women are allowed to have more power! Women are more powerful than men because they carry children!" I knew the coach was well-intended but his pep talk made my skin crawl. On Day 5 I called the lab for an update. An assistant said my results weren't ready yet because "we're busy assessing our patients." How strange: I wasn't sure if she meant the embryos themselves were her patients. Perhaps she did. That afternoon I got a call back: I had one early blastocyst, Grade B, and a morula that wouldn't survive the thaw, and the third embryo had stopped developing altogether on Day 3. So they froze the blastocyst.

I loved knowing the frozen blastocyst was sitting there waiting to be transferred. My icy jewel, my future. I waited a month for my high progesterone to settle and then did the transfer. Everything was timed to sync with my natural cycle. That morning Dr. Nell was running behind schedule so I meditated in the waiting room. I'd started seeing a new counselor, privately. A man. Unfairly or not, I'd stopped trusting the counselor at the clinic: should a fox counsel hens in the henhouse? I suppose I liked the male attention but also I'd grown to dislike confiding in a mother about my woes. The double bind: while I still had hope of becoming pregnant, perhaps in the next two weeks, it felt awkward to talk about giving up, eternal childlessness. I was too superstitious. And how could I grieve sincerely knowing there was still a chance I might soon be immensely happy? Half-grief, forestalled grief, was a kind of hell. To make it more bearable we focused on things like grounding oneself in the body, meditation. He mentioned the hara point, beloved of many traditions including Zen Buddhism. "It's about two inches below the belly button and then two inches inside the belly. Put your attention there." "Oh," I replied, snow-blind, "you realize that's the point of conception in a woman's body. Where humans are conceived." When I was in the chair for the transfer the doctor asked, kindly, "Are you all right? You're very quiet today." All the sadness in the world fell through the ceiling. "I'm OK," I lied. I passed the paperbark tree on the way to my car but didn't even touch it. In the parking spot reserved for Medical Practitioners Only I noticed a Bentley.

When I refused to use Zovirax for a cold sore on my lip, saying it wasn't suitable for pregnant women, my sister sighed and told me I was an idiot. After I ate some cold chicken salad from a bain-marie I was pierced with guilt lest I'd given myself food poisoning and compromised the baby. Day in, day out, my nipples were burning. Come Day 28 there were no signs of bleeding. *Hope.* Hope sharpened to *need.* I did the pregnancy test in the morning—a nightmare, Rebecca had to tap my vein while the needle was in place, tap tap tap, to encourage blood flow. Ten thousand hours later the nurse called and said, "We thought it might have been different because we hadn't heard from you but I'm sorry, it's negative." That night I took a Valium and watched back-to-back episodes of *Agatha Christie's Poirot.* Those mysteries were always solved. It was impossible to imagine the Belgian detective happy running after children.

By now a private equity-owned clinic in Sydney had floated on the stock exchange and become the world's first listed IVF company. Financial commentators said it had a great business model.

My period did arrive a couple of days later and I went straight into a new cycle. "I want to firebomb that place," said one of my friends. My donor was a prince and a gentleman. I let him know each pregnancy test how I'd fared and he always responded promptly with an encouraging message of support. My mother assured me she wished me well, "There's nothing I can do but I wish you all the very best, really, I mean it." Another friend—who is not Catholic and who had lost her first child at nine days old—gave me her picture of Piero della Francesca's *Madonna of Parturition*, a Renaissance portrait of the Virgin Mary, heavily pregnant, flanked by angels, her hand resting on her gown, split open, a holy lapis lazuli blue. So beautiful. I taped that to my wall. One thing I found consoling was a message from a friend who—completely pro-choice—said each encounter between a sperm and egg was magical, brief or not. "Bathe in love, mourn in love if necessary, thank the spirits for even a micro-moment of passing through." I confessed my fear of the abyss to my sister, who said I needed to start preparing.

But what if my period hadn't arrived? What if the test had been positive? My whole life would have changed. Just like that. I would have held my breath, warding off miscarriage, and at the same time every day would have been a joy. Morning sickness? Joy—I insisted. A child was a cure for nausea. My accountant had advised I shouldn't sell my apartment and move to a bigger place unless I knew exactly where I stood—so I could have gone ahead with that. A new place with a room for the baby. A new suburb because I couldn't afford to stay where I was. I would have opened my Hope Chest and pinned an embroidered wall hanging of colorful animals above the cot. Strung up paper garlands in the shape of butterflies and swallows. Run as fast as I could out of limbo.

There was another way out of limbo. The dark and rocky path. I made the decision that I would only try two more egg collections and do as many transfers as there were viable embryos. It was extremely hard to nominate my own breaking point and I did give myself a sneaky back-door which was something like "Well, see how you feel at the time." But now the abyss was ripped from the ever-receding horizon and fixed in place. *Crawl along that dark and rocky path.* My doctor raised the unironic possibility that I may have a high level of Natural Killer cells, the main immune cell-type found in the uterus, and that I may be rejecting the embryo in the same way my immune system would fight off cells not recognized as myself, such as infections or cancer. There were tests the clinic could run—either a blood test or a uterine biopsy or both. She advised studies so far had demonstrated an "association" between high Natural Killer cells and infertility but a causal relationship had yet to be established. *Yet*, I heard her *yet*: the science was so new. One more blood test didn't seem too onerous so I agreed to do that. Meanwhile the cycle was proceeding at the regular pace: injections, blood tests, scans. I was exhausted. Bone-tired. Knackered. *They shoot horses, don't they?* For the first time I forgot one of my nightly injections and woke at 5 a.m. in a panic, berating myself for this sloppiness. Why did you forget? Have you lost faith that things will work out? My sister picked me up from the egg collection. This time, after my fourth general anesthetic in the space of seven months, I needed to go on a drip before I was allowed to leave because of low blood pressure. The results of that penultimate cycle were disappointing. Of the eight eggs collected six were injected with sperm but overnight only one embryo showed signs of fertilization. That lone embryo developed strongly until Day 3—it looked as good as it could be, Grade A—and Dr. Nell recommended we transfer straightaway rather than wait until Day 5 because we were only monitoring one embryo. When I looked at my inner moonscape on the ultrasound screen and saw the tiny white speck land on my uterus I was surprised to hear the doctor say, "That's the baby." *The baby.* I loved her for saying "the baby." My not-yet-baby was real to her. I wasn't entirely alone. Maybe the doctor would be the only person in the world who would ever refer to my baby. I thought it generous.

A week later the Natural Killer cells test came back with a bad result: a high level of both the number of cells and their activity. I was with my sister and her two little girls in a café when the doctor called. I stepped outside. I was told I could begin the protocol immediately: a prescription was ready at the clinic for me to pick up. Treatment would involve me artificially suppressing my immune system for a period of three months. I would take a steroid, prednisone, and also a blood-thinning agent, Clexane.

—What are the side effects?
—The rate for cleft palate in the baby increases from one in 1,000 to three in 1,000.
—And for the mother?
—An increased chance of high blood pressure and high blood sugar.
—My friend went manic after she took steroids for an ear problem.
—Well, I don't know about that . . .
—When I took the test I was run down, I didn't have the flu but I'd finished fighting one off. Could that have spiked my immune activity?
—Possibly.
—Can I retake the test now?
—No, the reading would be off. We'd have to wait until next month.
—On the Internet I read that this Natural Killer cell therapy is controversial. What's the evidence?
—It's very new. There's not really enough evidence to show the benefits of treatment outweigh the down-

sides of doing it. It's up to you. The script is there if you want it.

—Can I think about it and let you know tomorrow?

—Yes, that's fine.

Artificially suppress my immune system for three months? I let the tears fall. When I reported back to my sister she frowned and said, "Where does this stop? It's too much stress on your body. I hate to say it but the main thing is the age of your eggs so any extra hope is marginal." I decided to hold off and retake the test.

During that two-week wait I flew up to Thursday Island in the Torres Strait to do some research for a script. The Torres Strait lies between the far north tip of Australia and Papua New Guinea. The doctor had said it was OK to fly and I figured the length of the longest leg in the air—Sydney to Cairns, three hours—was manageable. My friend, a leading corporate lawyer, rigorous and hardheaded, had strongly advised me against long-haul flights after she suffered a miscarriage herself shortly after one such long trip. "I'll never know if that was the cause," she said. "But you don't want to risk it." From Cairns I flew to the tiny airport on Horn Island—a pit stop before taking the ferry over to Thursday Island—and learned my luggage had gone missing. Stupidly, I'd packed away my medication—my progesterone pessaries—rather than carry it in my handbag. So when I arrived at my hotel I asked the receptionist to call the local pharmacy to check if they carried the pessaries. They didn't. Then she called the dispensary at the hospital—and I was in luck. I made my way there and arrived close to 5 p.m. when the dispensary was due to close. I presented myself to Emergency, extremely apologetic, feeling like a complete fool. *Princess!* No one else was waiting. I was informed the doctor was in with a patient. Tick-tock. What if the dispensary closes before the doctor can see me? I went to the desk and assured them, really, it would only take a minute for someone to write out a script. Finally the doctor, a woman who looked in her late twenties, emerged from a room. "We treat sick people here," was the first thing she said to me. I made my case as best I could. Outside came the sound of a chopper approaching. "Those are my patients," said the doctor. They were bringing in cases from the outer islands—who knows what? Machete cuts, croc bites, broken limbs. Anyway, she wrote me a script and I left with my pessaries hidden in a brown paper bag.

While I was up there I got my period. I confided to one of the Islander women that I was doing IVF. Her mother had adopted out her first child to an infertile couple. Across all the islands and among those Islanders living on the mainland the practice of traditional adoption was—and is—common. Widespread. Both married couples and single mothers adopt out. And for all sorts of reasons, not only helping those who are infertile. There is no stigma. The adoption takes place within extended family so link to kin and culture is preserved. I read a report that said "people are considered greedy if they have too many children and do not share them with others. The underlying principle of Torres Strait Islander adoption is that giving birth to a child is not necessarily a reason for raising the child." A clinic on the island would almost certainly go bankrupt.

The results of my second Natural Killer cell test came back. Both my levels—amount and activity—were now normal. I was relieved—and dismayed. Dismayed to realize that I had so narrowly escaped such an aggressive treatment. I asked Dr. Nell to bring my results to the attention of the in-house lead researcher and she later advised that the clinic would in future refine its advice about when to take the test.

To prepare for the abyss I tried to kill my baby. I defaced the little darling, removed its eyes, eye sockets too (pity the poor mother in Chernobyl whose baby was born with no eye sockets). I shrank and gnarled its limbs. I laid my umbilical cord around its neck like a noose. But it never worked. The childling was always resurrected, smiling, perfect.

Whenever people asked "How are you?" by way of social nicety I lied through my teeth. "Not too bad," I'd say. Or "Swings and roundabouts." At least I didn't say "Fine, thanks." Or "A livid scar cuts across my very being."

One morning I got up early to watch the World Cup final. Germany vs. Argentina. Looking out of my window, high on the hill, I saw that the entire valley of houses and apartments ringing the beach had vanished in a whitish fog, a sea mist. That happened sometimes, maybe twice a year. Germany beat Argentina in the dying minutes of extra time. I liked how Lionel Messi conducted himself. He didn't pretend. He wasn't thinking, We played well, we did our best. You could see the snub blade of defeat, under his ribs. Even when he went up on the dais to accept a trophy for best player of the tournament he didn't crack a smile. Something deeply meaningful to him had been lost. He—and his team—were truly defeated.

A friend very gently asked, "How's the other going?," discreetly referring to my IVF. I told her I was about to begin another cycle, "probably my last." She reached under the table and pulled a present from a large bag. It was an Aboriginal painting in a muslin wrap. "I'm glad to hear that. Here—you can have this on loan for as long as you like. It's a fertility painting, it has magical powers." I was so touched by this kind gesture. "I conceived my children with it in the room and I'd love you to have it." I tried not to cry. She tried not to cry. We smiled through our tears. Unspoken: her first child had died in utero at five months.

I asked the doctor if for this last cycle we could increase my Gonal-f dosage from 300 to 350 IU. A last hurrah. She agreed. But on the night I was due for my first injection I got cold feet. I'd read somewhere about high doses affecting egg quality—and I also got nervous about over-stimulation. So I only took 300 IU. The next day Dr. Nell assured me 350 IU wasn't considered especially high and I should be fine at that dose if I wanted. Snow fell in the night, it stormed. At my first scan I had nine large follicles and the nurse commented, "You're responding well this cycle." Nine eggs were collected. Six were injected with sperm and showed signs of fertilization. This time, by Day 5 I had two blastocysts. One Grade A blastocyst and a "very early blastocyst." The "very early blastocyst" was looked at by two scientists and judged to be on the wrong side of the borderline for freezing. The doctor asked if I'd like to transfer both embryos. I dreaded twins—highly unlikely—but couldn't face discarding a blastocyst so agreed to transfer both. When the image of the first magnified blastocyst came up on the monitor the doctor said, "There's the baby, see that clump of cells at nine o'clock?" After the transfer I went to the acupuncturist. I tried everything. *But did I? Did I really?*

I felt it—the twinge of implantation. I actually felt it.

Good morning, babies. I had the exquisite pleasure of greeting my babies-to-be each day. I was hopeful and shameless.

I ran into an acquaintance on the street. He was in the mood for a chat.

—How's things?

—Hard. With the IVF.

—I heard you were doing that. How many tries did you do?

—Two IUI's and six egg collections plus transfers.

—That's hard.

—Yes.

—Well, I have friends who did it twenty times and in the end they had a child. It was a real victory. It's worth it if you keep going. Are you going to try again?

—Probably not. I don't really want to talk about it.

—I have a picture of their kid. Do you want to see it?

—No.

—There's a guy who went to Thailand, a rich Japanese guy, and he had fifteen children. Used surrogates.

—He wanted to father fifteen children?

—He said he needs them.

—Oh.

—Having a kid isn't always that great. My son hardly ever calls me. So with the IVF—

—Sorry, I don't want to talk about it.

That night I had a horrible dream in which I told a woman, a mother of four, that my final attempt didn't work. "It's a heartbreaking pity, a heartbreaking pity," she said. And she kept repeating, "It's a heartbreaking pity" with a sliver of glee. "What a heartbreaking pity." I shrank from her mummy-*schadenfreude*.

I felt so sad when I had to tell Elsie that qcumber was spelled "cucumber." In other words, the world does not make sense.

We talked about her birthday cake. We could make a marshmallow cake. "And a flower cake, a remote control cake, a sofa cake, and a shoe cake," she added.

My pregnancy test fell just before Father's Day. I knew this because *The Morning Show* on the TV in the waiting room was devoted to a Father's Day special. I thought about the Taoist parable of a man who wouldn't be angry if an empty boat collided with his own skiff but if he saw a man in the boat then he would shout and be angry at that man. I'd long understood it to mean that if you were hit by empty circumstances then there was no cause for anger—fate, so be it—and you should apply this same monkish acceptance to those circumstances in which you could identify whom or what had hit you. But in fact, no. The parable goes on to say that if you can empty your own boat crossing the river of the world then no one will oppose or seek to harm you. It was hard then and it's hard now, emptying the boats.

Rebecca asked me if I'd done a test at home. No.

—Have you had a bleed?

—No.

—I don't want to be a Negative Nancy but sometimes the progesterone can stop you getting your period.

She took my blood. Careful, gentle. As I was leaving I stopped by the door.

—Thank you. I don't think I'll be seeing you again. Thanks for all your help. You were great.

My eyes flushed with tears, hers too.

—It's been my pleasure.

Reprieve or delight, reprieve or delight. While waiting for the nurses to call I tried to fool myself with a win-win outcome. I'd arranged to spend the day with my sister. When the phone rang I picked it up as if it were hot to the touch. And learned I was pregnant. I can't remember exactly how the nurse phrased it, something like, "It's a positive result but it's not clear. You have an hCG level of 10.5, which is very low. Your progesterone is 75, which is good. You'll need to come back in for another test on Monday."

Her news was confounding. I knew the hormone hCG (human chorionic gonadotropin) was produced by the embryo and measured in a pregnancy test but I didn't realize the test could be unclear.

—Well, what would you call a good level of hCG at this stage?

—75.

—And what level would be called a negative pregnancy result? Zero?

—No, 2.

—In your experience does someone with as low a level as mine have a viable pregnancy?

—Not usually, but we can't rule it out.

My sister wanted to know the result. I said, "I have a very complex answer to a simple question." We were in disbelief. She turned to Dr. Google and on a bulletin board found a woman who said she had an initial hCG level of 10.5 and then went on to have a child. *Hope.*

I called my doctor. Asked for clarification.

—If we wait over the weekend it will declare itself, we want to see the hCG level rise. Keep up the pessaries.
—What would you be happy with, level-wise?
—I'd be happy if it got to 25. But I should let you know it could be a biochemical pregnancy.
—What's that?
—It's when there's a positive result, there was implantation, but it might not be viable. Still, fingers crossed, this is the best result we've had so far.
—OK, I'll work on it . . .

There was nothing I could do except wait. It snowed all weekend. On Monday morning I woke to find the whitish sea mist had filled the valley. I went for a walk along the cliff tops and marveled that the ocean—flat, calm—was covered in a layer of snow or perhaps had turned entirely to snow. White, gently undulating, all the way to the horizon.

That afternoon the second pregnancy test came back negative. It was as if I were in the path of an oncoming vehicle and just before the moment of impact I vanished. I went to bed and sobbed until I was exhausted. Felt no reprieve, only despair. My snuffling tears—as a response—seemed hopelessly inadequate. I was thinking: I will never meet that little person. I didn't move for a long time. Then I called my sister, who offered to come over and collect me. "Oh darling," she said, "I'm so sorry." My next call was to Dr. Nell. Her tone was measured, kind. I tried to match it.

—I'm six for six fails. What should I do?

—Well, while you're still giving me blastocysts there's a possibility. I don't know how you are financially . . .

—I'm OK. It's my mental and physical health that's a wreck.

—Yes, you always told me this would be your last go. Is it because we got close this time that it's harder?

—That positive result threw a spanner in the works. I mean, what are the odds for me? A near miss is still a miss.

—With a Day 5 blastocyst there's a 40 percent chance.

—But I've transferred blastocysts . . . that figure doesn't seem right. Is that for women of all ages?

—Yes.

—Then what are the real odds?

—It's hard to say.

—What would you do if you were me?

—I think you should try again and if it doesn't work then that's the end. Unless you want to consider a donor egg.

—That's not an option for me now.

—Well, I'd try once more. Why don't you think about it. Give me a call if you have any questions.

My sister was frustrated that the doctor had suggested trying again.

—If you were in the natural world you wouldn't have even known about that positive result! It's only because you're doing IVF that you even know! You need to find another way to be happy. And if you really want a baby then use a donor egg. That's the only way it's going to happen for you.

—I don't want a stranger's egg.

—My friend got a huge thick file about her South African donor. She knows everything.

—I bet they don't run checks on the background. Anyway, I don't think I could ask a woman poorer than me for her body parts. Makes me uneasy.

—I'd do it for you, when I finish breastfeeding.

—You would?

—But only if you build up your strength. You need to be strong to carry a baby.

—I'll think about it.

—Good. Maybe now you'll do what I'm always telling you.

I drank half a bottle of Scotch and spent the night laid out dead on her sofa.

A few days later I wrote to ask the doctor a very specific question that I hadn't thought—or dared—to ask before: In the last year, what percentage of women my age at the clinic had taken home a baby using their own eggs? Her answer: 2.8 percent for 44-year-olds, 6.6 percent for

43-year-olds. I wish I could have known what the exact figures were for women my age producing five-day Grade A blastocysts but that number wasn't at hand.

What to do? What to do? *Where does this stop*?

My inner compass went berserk. Should I try one last time with my own eggs, transfer another blastocyst? But remember: a near miss is still a miss. So near and yet so far. Quixotic. Dame Errant. I have tried, I have tried. And could I really take my sister's egg and my friend's sperm and make a baby? Or was that a little too *Frankenstein*, too much? Did I sincerely believe that childling was meant-to-be? And could I bear to stay in limbo for months while I waited for my sister to finish breastfeeding? And what if something happened to her during the egg collection, what if something went wrong? Around and around. I became immaterial. I had to hold myself back from vanishing between the tiles on the bathroom floor, from slipping through the typeface. It was hard to give up, truly hard to give up the struggle. The struggle itself had been *sustaining*. "This time I'm not lucky" was a hard thing to say.

I don't remember the exact moment—I'm not sure there was an exact moment—but I resolved to stop everything.

In the distance I heard a loud rumbling crack.

"The boys love you," said my sister. "You're an important part of their lives." I was grateful for this consolation. She was the first person I told about my decision to stop. Dearest sister, who had been my steadfast companion through the long treatment, who had seen me cry more times in the last couple of years than at any other time of my life. Telling people was a way of fixing my decision. Marking my grave. My parents were kind. My friends too. Some of the mothers cried—tried not to cry and failed—we pretended not to cry together. *Not alone, not alone.* A friend said—rightly, with compassion—"Darling, you're in peril." Another friend said, "I've seen the scar on your back, it's enormous, you shouldn't even be alive. Be grateful for the life you have. I never knew how you could even *talk* with all those drugs you put in your body." I told her I was thankful she'd said that because I didn't want to feel like I was wimping out by giving up. "Oh my god, that's crazy."

Sometimes—with people who didn't know the whole story—the conversation went like this:

—I've decided to stop treatment. It didn't work.
—You can always adopt.
—I'm at the end of my journey.
—Oh.

Shopworn maybe, but that's the way I phrased it: I've reached the end of my journey.

I bought some extravagant presents for my donor and took him out to lunch. We raised a glass to "the brilliant and beautiful concept that didn't work." I loved him.

Even after I told everyone there was a part of me that still couldn't fathom it.

In my heart of hearts I always knew this, it wasn't a revelation: I have to save myself.

So keep writing. Stay near. Capture these strong feelings before they are blanketed by time.

Soon after stopping I was haunted by the IVF. All the Googling I'd done about pregnancy-related topics came back in the form of advertisements for things like Clearblue pregnancy detectors or maternity clothes. I took care not to expose myself to painful situations and made a mental note to avoid grocery shopping at 3:30 p.m. which was also school pickup time when the streets were running with kids. I expect I'll need to manage the terrain in this way for quite some time. Most of the baby things I'd collected I gave away. There were moments when I wanted to take my coffee cup and hurl it against the wall, moments that flickered within a deepening acceptance. My health was a ruin. I was totally worn down, worn out. My skin was bad and so were my hips. It could just be a function of my age but my physiotherapist said she sees a lot of women doing IVF for hip pain. She thinks the hormonal changes exacerbate pain in the joints and ligaments. One of my ovaries, about two months after my last egg collection, was uncomfortable and twice the size it was before treatment. There are cysts that weren't there on my initial ultrasound. I was worried about some sort of permanent damage but Dr. Nell advised the size of the ovaries naturally rose and fell depending on where I was in my cycle. That made sense—but I continue to harbor a small fear that in the future I might be unpleasantly surprised by some latent side effect of all the medication and surgeries. I did ask for copies of my medical records just in case.

I reminded myself that since I'd been prepared to be a single mother, since I'd so ardently wanted to change my life, I must also have divined an access to some tremendous reservoir of energy that would have made these things possible. My wish: it was a reservoir and not a mirage.

On the afternoon of my 45th birthday I went over to visit my sister and the little girls. Elsie, age 3, insisted we play a game. I had to lie down and pretend to be asleep. She came into the room calling out, "Wake up! It's your birthday!" In her hands was a large cardboard box which she solemnly passed to me as a present. "Oh, a present! Oh, what is it? What could it be?" I slowly, slowly opened the box. Her eyes widened with delight. Inside were some pieces of a pink jigsaw puzzle. "It's a box of babies!" said Elsie. She and her baby sister were now sharing a bedroom and so Elsie was obsessed by all things baby. We played with the jigsaw babies for a long time and I did not flinch. That would have been unthinkable a year ago. I was suffused with a burning tender love for that astonishing girl.

What I try to hold onto—now that the treatment has failed—is a commitment to love widely and intensely. *Tenderly.* In ways I would not have previously expected. *I* to *You*; *I* to *We*; *I* to *This.* To unshackle my love from the great love I wanted to give my own child.

After the avalanche, the bare face of the mountain. Under the sun and the moon.

Sydney, January/November 2015